SalonOvations'
Shiatsu
Massage

SalonOvations' SHIATSU MASSAGE

by
Erica T. Miller

© 1996 Milady Publishing Company
(a division of Delmar Publishers)
3 Columbia Circle, Box 12519
Albany, New York 12212-2519

NOTICE TO THE READER

Cover design: D. Dupras

Milady Staff:
Publisher: Catherine Frangie
Acquisitions Editor: Marlene McHugh Pratt
Production Manager: Brian Yacur
Project Editor: Annette Downs Danaher
Art/Design Production Coordinator: Suzanne McCarron

Photographs: Andy Sears, Correlations Inc.
Illustrations: Accurate Art Incorporated

Copyright © 1996
SalonOvations
(a division of Milady Publishing Company)
3 Columbia Circle, Box 12519
Albany, New York 12212-2519

Printed in the United States of America
Printed and distributed simultaneously in Canada

Library of Congress Cataloging-in-Publication Data

Miller, Erica T.
    SalonOvations' shiatsu massage by Erica T. Miller.
      p.   cm.
    Includes bibliographical references and index.
    ISBN 1-56253-264-2
    1. Acupressure. I. Title.
    RM723.A27M55 1995
    615.8'22—dc20
                      95-18511
                      CIP

Dedication

During the preparation of this book, I had the opportunity once again to visit the Japan Shiatsu College in Tokyo. I met with Mrs. Matsuko Namikoshi (Toru's wife), also a renowned expert instructor in *Shiatsu* Therapy and codirector of the school. I was saddened by the news that in mid-1994 Mr. Toru Namikoshi passed away.

This book is being dedicated to the Namikoshi family, three generations who have built and maintain the relevance of *Shiatsu* as an important allied health therapy. I have chosen to dedicate this book to them because of the training I received in Japan during the years I was living and working there.

I believe all practitioners of modern *Shiatsu* owe a great deal to Mr. Tokujiro Namikoshi who worked so hard to bring awareness of this specialty to the modern world. Mr. Namikoshi was born in Kagawa prefecture in Japan on November 3, 1905. At an early age his family moved to the northernmost island of Japan, Hokkaido. Due to the move to this very cold climate from a much more temperate one, his mother began to have acute, chronic rheumatism of the joints. He and his sisters and brothers would rub and press on their mother to help relieve her pain. She seemed most impressed with Tokujiro's technique and her praise of him led him to a continuing interest and career in massage.

His massage expertise grew and he began developing his *Shiatsu* techniques. He opened a school in Hokkaido in 1925 and it prospered. By 1940 he had opened another school in Tokyo. He worked and pioneered until the Japanese Ministry of Health and Welfare finally recognized *Shiatsu* and his Japan Shiatsu College and licensed it. (It wasn't until 1964 that the government recognized *Shiatsu* separately from massage.) All during that time and since, Namikoshi and his eldest son, Toru continued to work, teach, and expand the knowledge of *Shiatsu* throughout not only Japan but also the rest of the world. Toru published several English texts on the subject and traveled extensively in Europe, the United States, and Canada, training.

Tokujiro is now more than ninety years old and is still practicing, but the banner of management has now been passed on to Toru's son Takashi who is the director of the school and who plans to continue spreading the true Namikoshi Method of *Shiatsu* to the world. The school is located on the same site in Tokyo as it was originally because Tokujiro

v

insists that this specialty must continue on eternally from the same beginning. The Japan Shiatsu College offers year-round training for those desiring to become true experts in this field. We thank you for your courage, dedication, and hard work. For more information, contact: Japan Shiatsu College, 2-15-6 Koishikawa, Bunkyo-ku, Tokyo 112, Japan, Tel. 03-3813-7354.

Contents

Preface

Why is there a need for a book on *Shiatsu*? I wrote this book because *Shiatsu* is gaining popularity in America as a therapy in the beauty industry and even for home. In stores across America you now see "*Shiatsu* this" and "*Shiatsu* that," some giving the impression of curing a problem, some just gadgetry. I was originally exposed to *Shiatsu* more than twenty years ago, and I never thought it was a word I should have trademarked for products to be developed in the future. Perhaps *Shiatsu* will eventually become a generic term to represent all pressure-related therapies, in much the same way as Kleenex represents tissues or Xerox represents copy.

I wrote this book from a very different standpoint than other books in existence on the subject, that is from a beauty standpoint, not as a curative therapy for ailments. Every book that I have ever read concentrates on "fixing health problems." I believe that we are not only NOT licensed to cure, we don't even need to worry about that. Why can't we beauty practitioners be happy performing treatment for the sake of beauty and wellness enhancement instead of "curing" things? I believe in many ways we have gone far overboard in our treatments, leaning too much to the medical when we don't need to and legally can't anyway. This book, I hope, will be a first in demonstrating a modality of treatment that has a viable place in our armament of treatment from a positive, legal, and limited scope.

I have heard that I'm considered at this time to be the esthetic industry's top expert in *Shiatsu*. If this is the case, I feel you should know why. I have been teaching *Shiatsu* in America since 1976. Prior to that time, I was living and working in Japan as an esthetician for a cosmetic company called Kanebo Cosmetics. I went into the esthetic field after searching for a way to work in a Japanese company and polish my simultaneous interpreting abilities as my goal at that time was to work at the United Nations as an interpreter. I was trained in the Namikoshi method during my stay in Japan and began to teach it in other countries while working for this company. I enjoyed it, saw the benefits, and realized it would be of interest to estheticians in the United States as well.

Soon after my return to America I had my first opportunity to demonstrate the technique to a small group of estheticians at the All-Texas Beauty Show for Ron Renée and the Aesthetician International Association. The response was overwhelming, and I was hired to teach around the country. So since 1976 I've been married to this therapy, and I still have great demand for classes in this subject. In fact, the demand for classes has actually grown. (By the way, I never went back to interpreting due to my love for the esthetics field.) I'm definitely a staunch believer in *Shiatsu* from a treatment and business standpoint, and I hope you will find it just as exciting as I have. If you're ever in one of my classes I hope you'll let me know how you liked the book and my philosophy behind it. *Shiatsu* is a great subject and I hope you will study it further. Thank you for your interest in reading this book!

About the Author

Erica T. Miller is an internationally acclaimed educator with world-class qualifications and expertise. As a CIDESCO Diplomate and International Examiner, Ms. Miller is a founding member of NCA/CIDESCO USA, Liaison Committee Chairman for the Esthetics Equipment and Manufacturer's Alliance (EMDA) of the American Beauty Association (ABA), and was named one of the five most prominent women in American esthetics by *Salon News* magazine. She is listed in more than five *Who's Who in America* books, is a former associate publisher/editor of *Aesthetics World* magazine, has authored more than 300 articles in national publications, served as beauty director for the Neiman Marcus Greenhouse, and is the nation's best-known expert on *Shiatsu*. She is a graduate of Shaw College of Beauty in London. In addition to her esthetics expertise, Erica speaks fluent Japanese, having majored in Japanese at Sophia University, Naganuma Language School, and the Simultaneous Interpreter Academy in Tokyo. She has served as an official interpreter for Japanese visitors to the United States including members of the Kyodo News Service and United Press International. As chairman and president for Correlations, Inc., a Dallas-based full-service esthetics training and distribution company, Erica develops training programs and products for the Dallas Training Center and travels the country teaching advanced courses in a number of esthetics-related subjects.

Acknowledgments

I wonder if most of you reading this book will ever take the time to read this page. Perhaps for me it's the most important page in the entire book. When I undertook the challenge to write the first book on *Shiatsu* from a beauty standpoint I had no idea what a project it would turn into. And as with all books, no doubt, I couldn't have accomplished this without the help, support, and guidance of so many people. I would first like to thank Cathie Frangie, the publisher at Milady who saw this as a viable and important subject for the American beauty industry today and for her trust in asking me to write it. I couldn't have done the book without the constant encouragement of my editors and the support staff of Milady Publishing Company. Ms. Marlene Pratt, my acquisitions editor and friend, helped me over and over again and spent hours on the phone and in person working through the book with me. Ms. Annette Downs Danaher was also so patient with me as I began to learn more about computers and producing a book than I thought I could do and for fixing all my mistakes!

At home in Dallas, my entire staff at Correlations was behind me encouraging me to stay home to write whenever I could. They supported me with their attitudes and hard work, their prayers and verbal encouragement. I particularly thank Mary Catheryn Wisely, Paula Dean, and Andy Sears for the practical help of reading, locating information, faxing, proofing, talking, advising, etc. And a very important friend and client supported me all the way through by serving as a personal reviewer—Ms. Christine McKinnon, owner of Christine's Esthetics. Her professional opinion really gave me the encouragement to believe I was on target with the content and presentation of the material.

Also, a special thank-you to the following people for their assistance and expertise in reviewing this manuscript:

Jane Kane, Kingston, NY
Nancy Phillips, Tolono, IL
Haleh Palmer, Schenectady, NY
Bob Lunior, Miami, FL

And finally, above all I must thank my Father in heaven who gave me the ability, wisdom, and discernment to put words to blank pieces of paper that will hopefully help you on an ongoing basis for a long time to come. I'm truly grateful for the unique opportunity to write this book for you.

CAUTION

The art and science of *Shiatsu* is based on ancient Chinese medical practices. This book is designed to provide the student of Shiatsu with as much knowledge as possible to understand the mechanisms whereby it is used in health, alternative medicine, and beauty. Most books on the subject concentrate on the healing powers of *Shiatsu*, whereas this book serves as a preventative health and beauty manual, not a guide to healing. Even though the reader may gain insight that may improve or correct a health condition, it is not the purpose of this book to do so. Accordingly, this book should not be substituted for the physician. Seek the services of any and all appropriate health practitioners when health issues are involved. The author and publisher expressly disclaim any responsibility for any adverse effects as a result of your use of the material.

Time Line
HISTORY OF SHIATSU

2500 B.C. — Practice of acupuncture believed to have begun before this date; documents from Egypt claim medical treatment of the hands and feet.

800 B.C.–A.D. 1000 — Caraka-samhita and Susta-samhita produced

5th Century B.C. — Empedocles sets forth that the universe is composed of four elements—fire, air earth, and water—with four matching bodily humors—blood, phlegm, yellow bile, and black bile.

460 B.C. — Hippocrates, the father of modern medicine, born in Cos, Greece.

206 B.C.–A.D. 221 — Han dynasty; *Golden Mirror* documents medical developments during this period, including moxa, acupuncture, and herbalism. Asclepiades uses massage, tonics, and fresh air as remedies for various ailments.

A.D. 280 — Wang Shu-ho, Chinese physician, proposes concept of diagnosis based upon pulse; health depended on harmonious balance of *ying* and *yang*.

458 — First introduction of medicine into Japan by Korean physician.

600 — Japan begins sending monks and physicians to study in China.

618–907 — Tang dynasty; great period in Chinese history; Chinese medicine prospers and interests physicians the world over.

860 — Bronze model showing specific points for insertion of acupuncture needles produced; forerunner of numerous models and charts.

984 — *Ishinho* produced; first existent Japanese medical documentation.

1400s — Invention of Gutenberg printing press and proliferation of documented works; Leonardo da Vinci's drawings of human anatomy.

1478 — *De Medicina*, based on Greek medicine methodology, published by Cornelius Celsus.

1595 — René Descartes develops theory that body is divided into two, the physical body and the mind.

1700 — *Golden Mirror* produced; documents medical developments during the Han dynasty.

EARLY 1830s — Marshall Hall first to use term *reflex action*.

LATE 1800s — Charles Darwin's theory of evolution.

1890s–1930s — Sir Henry Head and Sir Charles Sherrington confirm there is a link between the brain, spinal cord, and reflex pathways; 1909: Dr. William Fitzgerald and Dr. Edwin Bowers popularize the concept of zone therapy; 1932: Dr. Joe Shelby Riley refines Fitzgerald's theories. Other theories of this period develop into modern day reflexology.

1902 — Dr. Alfons Cornelius's book *Druck-punkte, or Pressure Points, Their Origin and Significance* published.

NOVEMBER 3, 1905 — Birth of Tokujiro Namikoshi, the Father of Japanese *Shiatsu.*

1913 — Dr. Kurakichi Hirata, a Japanese psychologist, adds horizontal zones to zone system.

1920 — Traditional Chinese therapy combined with Dr. Hirata's research to create *Shiatsu* as a uniquely Japanese treatment.

1930s — Eunice Ingham separates the body zones from their origins on the feet; concentrates on feet; develops what is known today as reflexology.

1932 — Sir Charles Sherrington wins Nobel Prize for work on reflex action.

1938 — Eunice Ingham's book *Stories the Feet Can Tell* published.

1940 — Namikoshi Institute of Shiatsu Therapy opens; the first institute devoted solely to *Shiatsu.*

LATE 1940s — Auriculotherapy (a system of acupuncture for the ears) is first introduced by Dr. Paul Nogier, from France.

1955 — Japanese Ministry of Health and Welfare recognizes *Shiatsu* as a valid treatment modality.

1960s — Dr. Kim Bong Han finds evidence of a series of ductlike tubes corresponding to the paths of traditional acupuncture

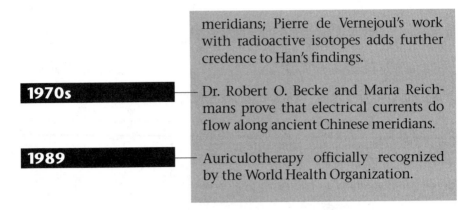

meridians; Pierre de Vernejoul's work with radioactive isotopes adds further credence to Han's findings.

1970s — Dr. Robert O. Becke and Maria Reichmans prove that electrical currents do flow along ancient Chinese meridians.

1989 — Auriculotherapy officially recognized by the World Health Organization.

PART I

THE HISTORY AND DEVELOPMENT OF SHIATSU

CHAPTER 1

Introduction to Shiatsu

Shiatsu, a Japanese term that directly translated means "finger pressure," represents a health and beauty therapy that has been used in numerous forms for more than five thousand years. This history is, of course, difficult to trace back, and that is not entirely necessary for this book. However, modern *Shiatsu* as we will study it has origins solidly placed in history. This author believes that the history emanating from the Orient provides the basic foundation for all subsequent adaptations of its traditional and original beginnings. But as with all things in history that are passed down from one generation to another, cross-cultural influences eventually crisscross to provide the modern therapies we use today.

Strains and developments of research come to us here in America not only from the Orient but also from Europe. The various techniques and concepts we currently use in massage therapy are an amalgamation of all the historical developments, and the individual naming and adaptations may often confuse the student of massage. We will touch on many of these adaptations; this is why aspects of history are critical to a clear understanding of what *Shiatsu* is all about.

Another aspect of the importance of the historical background and acceptance of *Shiatsu* lies in the simple fact that we can't necessarily prove scientifically and measurably how and why it works. The fact that *Shiatsu*, which originated from acupressure and acupuncture in India and China, has survived the test of time is good enough for those of us who have seen the results and proof of treatment effectiveness. Nevertheless, these results are often impossible to prove by any modern scientific measurements.

There is some empirical evidence of the physiological effects of *Shiatsu* but not enough to convince the established medical community of the curative and preventative benefits. Hence, *Shiatsu*, along with most forms of massage and holistic health practices, still falls into the category of an "alternative health practice." Furthermore, even though we in the beauty industry are not using *Shiatsu* for any medical application, it's still interesting and exciting to improve the health of our clients "by accident."

3

Without a clear understanding of some of the more salient points of the historical basis of *Shiatsu*, it is difficult for us to really understand why we would use it for any reason other than that it sounds exotic and probably feels good, when in fact it's slightly uncomfortable.

TARGET POINT

The word *Shiatsu* is of Japanese origin and means "finger pressure." The beginning history emanating from the Orient provides the basis for *Shiatsu* and all the various adaptations of it. This history, therefore, is very important.

As I will reiterate numerous times throughout the book, we are not using *Shiatsu* for the practice of medicine. However, the history of *Shiatsu* is purely medically based so we must delve into it for a better understanding of what this is all about. Then we'll more clearly understand what realistic effects we may expect in preventative health and beauty treatments. If I state that by doing *Shiatsu* in a full body treatment you can elevate the client's own physical sense of well-being, this means nothing unless you understand how and why it happens. The fact that this goes back to medical and surgical practices from ancient China carried on until today immediately lends credibility to the possibility of this effect, irrespective of the apparent lack of enough scientific proof.

TARGET POINT

The long history lends credence to the practice of *Shiatsu* and its therapeutic effects on the human body.

Another aspect of the history that further validates the claims we make today lies in some of the ancient religious practices in the Orient. In religious historical studies are found a number of interesting pictorial and papyrus documentation containing references to massage of the body and feet, to "touch" and its physiological effects on the well-being of the person as well as medical cures. We owe a lot to the early religious community worldwide for the documentation of early medicine.

TARGET POINT

Historical and religious historical papers and pictorials show us that this modality has been used for thousands of years.

Studies over the last fifty to seventy-five years have provided us with profound evidence of treatment effectiveness along with modern adaptations and variations of the ancient treatment principles.

HISTORY

India

It is believed that massage originated in India and China. It is further believed that the origins of Chinese herbal medicine along with acupressure and acupuncture actually began in India and Persia. We know that the ancient Indians worshiped many gods, one of whom was Vishnu who was represented by a view of the world on his feet. The concept was that the feet represent a microcosmic picture of the universe. Much of early Indian medicine was documented in the sacred writings called the Vedas.

Ayurvedic medicine, which we will discuss more thoroughly later, lasted until about 800 B.C. Ayurvedic medicine (meaning "science of life") is a system that combines natural therapies with a highly personalized approach to the treatment of disease. It places equal emphasis on the mind, body, and spirit and strives to restore the complete harmony of the three. From 800 B.C. to about A.D. 1000, called the Brahmanistic period, some medical treatises known as Caraka-samhita and Susta-samhita after physicians of the same name were produced. The theories contained in these documents remained the basis of Indian medicine until about the eighth century.

The Hindus believed that the body was comprised of three elements representing the entire universe. These elements were microcosmic representatives of the divine universal forces called spirit (air), phlegm, and bile. (The later humors of the Greeks coincide.) Health was based upon the harmony of the three. The phlegm represented the area of the body above the heart, the bile was between the heart and the navel, and the spirit was below the navel. (This will be modified somewhat in Chinese medicinal concepts.) The premise was that all functions of the body were based upon the interrelation of the three elements. In addition, Indian medicine also incorporated the use of between 500 and 760 known plants.

TARGET POINT

Indian medicine is based on three elemental forces: phlegm, representing the body above the heart; bile, representing the body between the heart and navel; and spirit, representing the body below the navel. These forces represent a microcosm of the entire universe and all that's in it.

China

The ancient Hindu and Buddhist monks are believed to have taken concepts of medicine to China. However, the *Nei Ching* (often called the *Classic of Internal Medicine*), the earliest canon of internal medicine by Huang Ti (the famous Yellow Emperor who died around 2598 B.C.), reportedly documents a medicinal system independent of any Indian influence. We know that acupuncture and other medical therapies may have begun as early as four thousand years ago. Most of the Chinese medical literature of old is based upon the *Nei Ching* and is still regarded with great respect.

Another work compiled around A.D. 1700, the *Golden Mirror*, documents the medical developments during the Han dynasty (206 B.C.-A.D. 221). This was the time of the greatest Buddhist and Hindu influence into China from India. At this time in history, most of the travel and educational influence from country to country was through the Buddhist monks. Chinese medicine may have originated in the northern part of China in the region of the Yellow River valley. Three primary therapies are documented as emanating at this time from this region: moxa, acupuncture, and herbalism.

TARGET POINT

Chinese medicine was based on three separate therapies: moxibustion, acupuncture, and herbal medicine.

Moxibustion. Moxibustion was a form of medical treatment, still practiced today. The area of the Yellow River valley at that time was fairly barren and consisted of small grasses and plants, including a plant called mugwort. The mugwort was dried, shredded, and placed in a small pile on the skin or over a thin stone and then set on fire to cause a drawing and disinfecting effect on body areas of injury or infection. The heat generated also gave physical relief to pain. This came to be called moxa.

TARGET POINT

Moxa was the burning of mugwort on the skin to draw out infection or relieve pain by heat.

Acupuncture. In addition to moxa, massage on certain strategic areas was provided to relieve pain and discomfort. This method of pain relief by massage became the basis of acupuncture for anesthesia, as well as the most serious form of medical treatment. Acupuncture, or needle insertion into the body at strategic points, is based upon a Chinese concept of the universe and all that's in it being either *yin* or *yang*. The *yang*, positive or male principle, is active and light and is represented by the heavens. The *yin*, negative or female principle, is passive and dark and is represented by the earth.

The human body, like matter in general, is also based upon *yin* and *yang* (later specific organs would also have a particular connection) and corresponding elements of wood, fire, earth, metal, and water. It is believed that in conjunction with this lies an energy pathway system of twelve vertical channels in the body that have corresponding points (which will be known in our study later as *Tsubo* or motor points) that link the whole body. These points along the channel form the basis of acupuncture as well as *Shiatsu*. Today we refer to this energy system as the "meridian system," which will all be discussed later in detail. Interestingly, anatomy was not known at this time, but it was believed that somehow this meridian system was correlated to the blood flow in the blood vessels and hence the pulse. The *Nei Ching* stated that the blood flowed continuously in a circle and never stopped. This eventually developed the doctrine of the pulse.

It is believed that another Chinese physician, Wang Shu-ho (approximately A.D. 280), proposed the concept of diagnosis based upon pulse and stated that the health of the body depended on the harmonious balance of the *yin* and the *yang*. A bronze model from around A.D. 860 shows hundreds of specified points for the insertion of the acupuncture needles and became the forerunner of numerous models and charts. The site of needle insertion is chosen to affect a particular organ or system, and the needle could be inserted at any number of corresponding points along the same or related meridian. The practice of acupuncture is believed to date from before 2500 B.C.

TARGET POINT

The Chinese concept of the universe was based on the balance between *yin* and *yang*. Yin, the female principle, represents dark, passive and equals earth. *Yang*, the male principle, represents light, active and equals heavens. Corresponding elements of wood, fire, earth, metal, and water have connecting areas on the human body.

TARGET POINT

The energy pathway system of the body has twelve longitudinal channels called the "meridian system." The corresponding points that link the system are the acupuncture points.

Herbalism. In contrast to the arid country of the north where moxa and acupressure massage proliferated, the southern region of China was rich in plants. The people began to use these various plants to make medicinal products for healing. They used the dry roots and stems of the plants along with the barks of various trees. This herbal medicine (which is called *Kanpo* in Japanese based on the Chinese written characters representing the Han dynasty) formed the basis of Chinese medicine that was eventually exported into Japan and Europe through the monks.

The combination of the three—moxa, acupuncture, and Chinese medicine—is still used today in the Orient and the rest of the world. The Han period was a great time in Chinese history, a prosperous flourishing time in which overland trade routes to Europe were developed. Another great and similar period in Chinese history was the Tang dynasty (A.D. 618–907). Chinese medicine prospered and interested physicians the world over.

TARGET POINT

Chinese herbal medicine comes from the southern region of China where many plants and grasses flourished.

Japan

It is believed that the first introduction of medicine into Japan was around the year A.D. 458 when a Korean physician settled in Japan. It wasn't until around the 600s, however, that Japan began to send physicians and monks to study in China, and this marks the real beginning of Chinese influence in Japan. The first and oldest existent Japanese medical documentation appears in the *Ishinho* (A.D. 984), a 30-volume work allegedly written by Tamba Yasuyori and based entirely on Chinese medicine.

For more than six hundred years all medical development in Japan was based upon earlier Chinese work and the theory of *yin* and *yang*. In fact, the first medical book published in 1528 was a Chinese work. Chinese medicine has been practiced in Japan ever since; however, the development of modern *Shiatsu* did not take root until the 1920s due to about two hundred-plus years of Western medical influences.

As Japan began to understand modern medicine in the 1500s Europe became the leading force for all Japanese medical developments. German medicine became the paramount influence from the mid-1800s until recently. As the concept of zone therapy and reflex reactions became popular in the late 1800s and early 1900s in Europe, interest was once again revived in Japan. In about 1913 a Japanese psychologist, Dr. Kurakichi Hirata, added another system of zones different from the Chinese vertical zones. These were horizontal zones where the body was divided into seven regions with twelve further refined zones in each region. It would appear that there was a lot of development around the world about this time and the discoveries were not necessarily interrelated.

Around 1920, the combination of traditional Chinese therapy began to combine with the research of Dr. Hirata. *Shiatsu* eventually became a uniquely Japanese treatment and the modern Father of *Shiatsu*, Tokujiro Namikoshi, is credited with the development and advancement of the technology. He opened the Japan Shiatsu College in 1940 as the first institute devoted solely to *Shiatsu*. In 1955, the Japanese Ministry of Health and Welfare finally recognized *Shiatsu* as a valid treatment modality along with Japanese massage called *Amma* and Western-style massage. Although there are now variations on the original Namikoshi method, the Nippon Shiatsu School is still the predominant methodology used the world over.

TARGET POINT

Chinese medicine entered Japan through Korea around 458 B.C. Later the *Ishinho* (A.D. 984), a 30-volume work written by Tamba Yasuyori, was based entirely on Chinese medicine.

TARGET POINT

In 1913 Dr. Kurakichi Hirata developed another system of zones similar to the Chinese, but these were seven horizontal zones with twelve zones within each of the seven larger ones.

TARGET POINT

Tokujiro Namikoshi is credited as being the Father of Modern *Shiatsu*. He began the Japan Shiatsu College in Tokyo in 1940 and finally achieved Japanese governmental acceptance in 1955.

EGYPT, GREECE, ROMAN EMPIRE

Some of the papyrus documents from Egypt claim medical treatment of the hands and feet as early as 2500 B.C. Of great interest is the fifth century B.C. when Empedocles set forth that the universe was composed of four elements—fire, air, earth, and water—which led to the doctrine of the four bodily humors: blood, phlegm, chole or yellow bile, and melancholy or black bile. Health was maintained by a balance of the four humors. This, of course, related very closely to the ancient Indian beliefs.

TARGET POINT

Empedocles (fifth century B.C.) set down a theory of the universe being composed of four elements—fire, air, earth, water—with four matching bodily humors—blood, phlegm, yellow bile, black bile. This is quite similar to Indian theory.

Later, Hippocrates (born in Cos, Greece, around 460 B.C.), the theoretical Father of Modern Medicine, was said to have studied massage and gymnastics (exercise) and left behind numerous recommendations on massage. He believed that disease was of natural cause and was heavily influenced by the inside as well as outside of the body. He believed in the healing power of nature and natural cures. He is, of course, best known for the charter of medical conduct known as the Hippocratic oath, still used today in graduating physicians from medical school.

Plutarch referred to the daily pinching treatment on Julius Caesar for his problems with neuralgia. Even Pliny, the great Roman naturalist, had himself massaged with various essences for his asthma. In the work *De Medicina*, a book printed in Florence in 1478 by Cornelius Celsus (based on Greek medicine methodology), references are made to the work of Asclepiades of Bithynia (around 120 B.C.) who used the typical Greek remedies of the day, including massage, poultices (similar to moxa), occasional tonics, fresh air, and corrective diet.

The documentable scientific evidence of anatomy perhaps really began with Galen, who discovered that the arteries contained blood and that the heart was the pump that caused the blood to move through the arteries but didn't realize that blood circulates throughout. After the fall of Rome, medical education and scientific development stagnated for a number of years.

TARGET POINT

Hippocrates believed that disease was of natural cause and should be treated naturally. He believed in the healing power of natural cures and is said to have recommended massage as a method of cure.

TARGET POINT

Greek history (written in *De Medicina* in 1478) going as far back as 120 B.C. suggests medical treatments that included massage and poultices (similar to moxa).

Throughout Europe medicine made little progress until the latter part of the fourteenth century, with perhaps the exception of Marco Polo (from Venice). He is said to have traveled China extensively and took great knowledge back to Europe, including evidence of massage.

MODERN HISTORY

It is said in some circles that modern medicine really began in Europe around the early 1400s after the invention of the Gutenberg printing press and the subsequent proliferation of documented works. By the time of Leonardo da Vinci anatomy and physiology had made great strides, including da Vinci's first drawings of human anatomy.

Then around 1595 a French philosopher, mathematician, and scientist, René Descartes, developed the theory that the physical body had to be divided into two, the physical body and the mind. This development perhaps slowed the progress of mind and body connection but helped the cause of scientific advancement in medicine. Progress continued, and in the late 1800s Charles Darwin promulgated the theory of evolution, which served to revolutionize medical science and subsequent breakthroughs. It was at about this point that many theories developed and grew that eventually resulted in modern-day reflexology.

TARGET POINT

Between the 1400s and 1800s in Europe scientific advances were documented including the charting of human anatomy by Leonardo da Vinci, separation of mind and body by René Descartes in 1595, and the theory of evolution by Charles Darwin in the late 1800s.

SUMMARY

Shiatsu's beginnings go back to China and India more than five thousand years ago. The historical development took Chinese medicine into Japan around 458 B.C. where it was further developed into the therapy we see today the world over. With time, the basic concepts of *Shiatsu* have evolved into other practices and methods with other names, but the foundations originally evolved from ancient India and China. Certain aspects of this meridian system and linking points may be difficult to prove scientifically, yet the effects have certainly passed the tests of time.

REVIEW QUESTIONS

1. Upon what is Ayurvedic medicine based?
2. Chinese medicine includes what three elements?
3. What is the meridian system?
4. For what is Hippocrates known?
5. When did Chinese medicine enter Japan?
6. What does the word *Shiatsu* mean?
7. What do *yin* and *yang* represent?

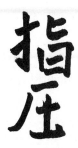

CHAPTER 2

The Development of Reflexology

We left off in chapter 1 around the 1890s in Europe for an important reason. Although *Shiatsu* was eventually to become popularized in the United States in the true Japanese form after the late 1950s, acceptance was hard and happened as a part of the European-to-American development of reflexology. Those specializing in *Shiatsu* treatment for the whole body have the erroneous tendency to think lightly of reflexology and relegate it to a minor version of *Shiatsu* that concentrates on the feet or hands. This couldn't be more mistaken.

By understanding the history and development of zone therapy to reflexology you will come to realize what a critical role reflexology played and still plays in the acceptance of the scientific and medical communities worldwide. It's important to understand this because it is this author's opinion that we owe the final emergence and acceptance of *Shiatsu* in America largely to the development and proliferation of reflexology.

TARGET POINT

Shiatsu continued to develop in Japan, but it was actually the European development of zone therapy and ultimately reflexology that eventually facilitated the popularization of *Shiatsu* in the United States.

EUROPEAN AND AMERICAN DEVELOPMENTS

It must be kept in mind that Western medicine, particularly American medicine, owes most of its history to Europe. Modern medicine in the early twentieth century didn't accept anything that couldn't be scientifically documented. The meridian system of acupuncture and acupressure could not be proven or demonstrated by any means acceptable to the Western medical community. Hence, Chinese medicine and all its practices were shunned in this country.

Reflexology is, of course, part of the same Chinese science as *Shiatsu*. As we explore European development, it's interesting to note how the same concept of medicine evolved into the many different applications we have today. In our study we will follow the development of this therapy from Europe to America and then back to Europe and the rest of the world.

TARGET POINT

Reflexology entered the United States before *Shiatsu* did.

Studies in Europe

In the early 1800s the brain and its functions began to be studied. In or around 1833, an English physiologist, Marshall Hall (1790-1857), was probably the first to use the term *reflex action* in demonstrating the difference in reflex actions of the brain and spinal cord. The concept of reflex action and pressure on the traditional Chinese meridian zones eventuated in a treatment known as zone therapy.

Neurological studies were also taking place in the 1890s and early 1900s by such well-known researchers as Sir Henry Head and Sir Charles Sherrington of England. The investigative development of neurology led to theories that neurologically connected the skin with organs. Head and Sherrington's work on the reflex action of the nervous system came to be taught in medical schools and confirmed that there was a link between the brain, spinal cord, and reflex pathways to control functions of the entire body. In 1932 Sherrington's work won him the Nobel Prize.

TARGET POINT

The science of neurology began to develop a direct connection between the brain, spinal cord, and other parts of the body. Dr. Marshall Hall (1790–1857) was the first to use the term *reflex action* in or around 1833.

At the same time, massage to reflex zones was being done in Germany by Dr. Alfons Cornelius. His book, *Druckpunkte, or Pressure Points, Their Origin and Significance* (1902) pointed out that pressure application (as in Chinese acupressure) incited various changes in the body, from stimulating muscular action to organ activity. The pressure points he used were believed to follow pathways along the nerves of the body. These pressure points were found on the body's surface as well as in the musculature. The important point to remember here is that all these scientists found that reflex stimulation in one area caused stimulation to other areas.

TARGET POINT

Many scientists found that reflex stimulation in one area of the body corresponded with stimulation in another.

Another important development in the science of zone therapy or reflex treatment is credited to the research of the American Dr. William Fitzgerald, who is perhaps considered the father of Modern Zone Therapy. He felt that direct pressure on certain areas of the body would produce an analgesic effect in a corresponding part. He systematized the body into the zones that reflexologists generally base their theories on today.

Another physician working with Fitzgerald was Dr. Edwin Bowers, and the concept of zone therapy became popularized by the two of them, although it's believed that much of their information came from previous European literature. This zone therapy was primarily designed for and demonstrated the anesthetic value of applying pressure in one area and then pricking or sticking a pin in another area without pain. Fitzgerald's body was divided into ten longitudinal zones.

It's interesting here to note that at about the same time in Japan Dr. Kurakichi Hirata (1913) was also developing a zone-based system but his were horizontal instead of the traditional vertical zones. There is, however, no literature to suggest a crossover in this research.

TARGET POINT

Dr. William Fitzgerald is the Father of Modern Zone Therapy.

Even with Fitzgerald's research, the subject of zone therapy was not generally accepted in America and only a few physicians followed him, one being Dr. Joe Shelby Riley. He believed so strongly in Fitzgerald's therapy that he researched and practiced his system and then continued to refine it. He developed and added more concepts of zones and points, including some reflex points on the ears.

Dr. Riley had a school in Washington, D.C., but often wintered in Florida. He had an assistant therapist there in the 1930s who would later make a profound dent in the history of zone therapy. Her name was Eunice Ingham. She would later go on and further develop this therapy into what is today known as reflexology. She separated the body zones from their origins on the feet.

She made several changes in the then current ideology and concentrated her efforts on the feet. It was her belief that instead of applying constant pressure to anesthetize, an alternating pressure could actually work to heal and stimulate the body to heal itself. After using the term of the day, zone therapy, she finally coined the word reflexology, which she used in her 1938 book *Stories the Feet Can Tell*. She charted the feet according to the zones and their effects on the rest of the body.

Today she is generally recognized as the founder of foot reflexology, and her foot charts are still widely used. Eunice Ingham died in 1974 after more than forty years of teaching and practicing. Her nephew Dwight Byers has continued her work along with other notable reflexologists such as Mildred Carter and Barbara and Kevin Kunz. The therapy has grown to include reflexology for the hands as well.

TARGET POINT

Eunice Ingham developed the concept of foot reflexology by separating the body zones from the feet around 1938. Her theories are the generally accepted method of treatment to this day, with further adaptations and advancements.

Back To Japan

Now let's go back to Japan for a moment. We left off with the development of the Nippon Shiatsu School of Tokujiro Namikoshi.

In the early 1950s he began to travel throughout the United States doing seminars and classes on *Shiatsu*. He also became quite well known for treating Marilyn Monroe and Joe DiMaggio. Dr. Namikoshi was responsible for the legislation in Japan that recognized *Shiatsu* as a viable science and ultimately developed a national licensing board. The Namikoshi system of *Shiatsu* still follows many of the original Chinese acupuncture points (*Tsubo*, motor points).

Other variations of *Shiatsu* are based upon different interpretations of the Chinese meridian system. Some of these include the method as taught by Wataru Ohashi, Jin Shin Jutsu developed in Japan by Jiro Murai, Zen *Shiatsu* by Masunaga, and Soku Shinjutsu. All of the various applications are quite similar.

ORIGINS: THE MERIDIAN SYSTEM

Since *Shiatsu*, acupressure, zone therapy, and reflexology all owe their origins to the ancient Chinese meridian system and acupuncture, it is, perhaps, interesting to note where acupuncture stands currently in scientific perspective.

TARGET POINT

Even though *Shiatsu* and reflexology are approached differently, they still owe their origins and allegiance to the same ancient Chinese meridian system concepts.

Acupuncture

As stated earlier, acupuncture is based on the concept of an energy pathway system in the body termed the meridian system. The twelve pathways are directly linked to specific internal organs and organ systems. It is said that there may be more than one thousand acupuncture (acupressure) points (*Tsubo* or motor points) in the body that can be stimulated to enhance its overall energy system. When special needles are inserted into the body they can help correct and rebalance the flow of energy and consequently restore health or relieve pain. The big question is whether this system is really there. The questions surrounding this have kept the scientific community leery of the therapy for decades.

Scientific Validation of the Meridian System

In the 1960s Dr. Kim Bong Han and a team of researchers in Korea attempted to prove the existence of meridians in the human body by using microdissection techniques. They allegedly found evidence of a series of fine ductlike tubes corresponding to the paths of traditional acupuncture meridians. These ducts appear to be different from the vascular and lymphatic systems that Western medicine has identified. They believe that the meridians themselves might exist within these ducts.

A French researcher, Pierre de Vernejoul, further researched the possibility of meridians by injecting radioactive isotopes into the acupoints and then into the blood vessels at random intervals.

The isotopes apparently didn't travel in the same manner, adding further credence to the theory that the meridian system is indeed a separate pathway system.

TARGET POINT

There has been scientific testing and evidence to prove the existence of the meridian system.

In addition, there have been numerous studies using electrical devices to measure the galvanic skin response (GSR) and further validate the existence not only of the meridians, but also of the heightened conductivity of the specific acupoints tested. Of great importance was the study sponsored in the 1970s by the National Institutes of Health. Under a grant Dr. Robert O. Becke and Maria Reichmanis, a biophysicist, were able to prove that electrical currents did indeed flow along the ancient Chinese meridians and that some of the points were also scientifically measurable.

TARGET POINT

Dr. Robert O. Becke and biophysicist Maria Reichmanis were able to prove that electrical currents could be measured and followed along the ancient Chinese meridians.

The World Health Organization has now recognized more than 104 conditions that can be treated by acupuncture. Furthermore, in 1989 the organization officially recognized auriculotherapy as a viable medical modality. Dr. Paul Nogier, a French physician, developed a system of acupuncture and acupressure for the ears shortly after World War II. He developed a system of thirty points on the ears, which when properly stimulated would neurologically affect other parts of the body. It is impressive to learn that the Chinese government has even accepted Dr. Nogier's work. He is now considered to be the Father of Auriculotherapy worldwide.

TARGET POINT

The fact that the development of auriculotherapy by a French physician has progressed so far that it is accepted by the Chinese government further shows the modern validity of this ancient science.

SUMMARY

We see that development of reflex action in the late 1800s led to the ultimate discovery in Europe and America of zone therapy. Zone therapy was promulgated as a result of the discovery of neurological connections between the brain, spinal cord, and other parts of the body and the system whereby a stimulus in one area could correspond directly to another area. As the concept of nerve zones became further developed, the feet as a central reflex zone were separated by Eunice Ingham in the 1930s and formed the basis of modern reflexology.

The late 1940s and early 1950s brought *Shiatsu* and auriculotherapy to the American shores and, combined with reflexology, served to create the basis of treatments still used today, all relating directly back to ancient China and the meridian system. In the opinion of acupuncturists, *Shiatsu* experts, and reflexologists there is no question about the existence of meridians and acupoints. Unfortunately, however, legislation in America still does not conclusively embrace these therapies.

Shiatsu and reflexology are still fighting for their place as viable allied health modalities. At the present time in most states *Shiatsu* and reflexology normally are performed by licensed massage therapists (in the states where licensing exists). Historically, all therapies based upon the Chinese meridian system are essentially medically based. However, it is perhaps best to leave any and all medical applications to the medical field and licensed acupuncturists.

For those of us in the allied fields of health and beauty, it is essential, if we are to be able to continue to use these modalities, that we do not cross over into the medical arena with our goals and claims. We legally treat healthy, albeit stressed, individuals, and our therapy is purely preventative in nature. In the next chapter we will discuss the meridian system and *Shiatsu* concepts in detail.

REVIEW QUESTIONS

1. From where did the term *reflex action* come?

2. What did English researchers Sir Henry Head and Sir Charles Sherrington contribute to the concept of reflex action?

3. Who developed the theory that pressure application incited various changes in the body?

4. Who is considered the Father of Zone Therapy?

5. Essentially, what is zone therapy?

6. With what is Eunice Ingham credited?

7. For what important legislation is Tokujiro Namikoshi responsible?

8. Do *Shiatsu* experts and reflexologists practice medicine?

9. Is there any validity to the concept of Chinese meridians?

CHAPTER 3

Total Harmony of *Ki*

The basis of *Shiatsu* and all forms of this ancient traditional Chinese healing practice lies in the concept of total harmony between humans and the universe. The term for this overall life force energy is called *Qi* or *Chi* in Chinese, Prana in Indian, and *Ki* in Japanese. The *Ki*, or universal energy, flows within the body through a pattern or matrix that links the body's vital organs with all the other body parts and the body to all environmental forces of nature. Without all aspects of nature and body being in harmony, the balance of *Ki* cannot be maintained.

The ancient Chinese made no specific distinction between the different body parts such as nerves, lymphatics, and blood vessels. They considered a system of life forces in the body that allowed people to breathe, think, exist. In Western medicine we have a detailed knowledge of anatomy, physiology, and chemistry but little knowledge of what actually makes it all work.

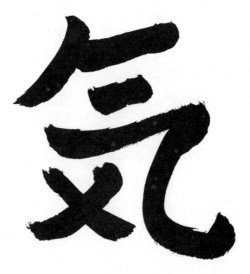

Chinese symbol for *Ki*. (Graphic by Lillian Sou.)

To the Chinese all the myriad things in heaven obey the law of *Ki* balance, from the sun rising to the wind and rain, from the outside to the inside, and from the inside to the outside. As complicated as it can be when studied in detail, it also provides a most interesting method of understanding how all life forces work together. To the oriental mind it's really a simple principle as far as health and well-being goes. When all elements of *Ki* are working in harmony, the body is healthy and full of energy, moods are better, the person is happy, and so it goes with all outside elements as well. In other words, the harmony of *Ki* provides the harmony of all aspects of the universe.

TARGET POINT

The question we normally ask is "how does it work?" Perhaps we should just ask, "does it work?" The concepts behind *Ki* evade Western logic.

YIN AND YANG

The harmony that is central to the understanding of traditional Chinese and Japanese philosophy, science, and culture lies in the balance of *yin* and *yang*, the well-known figure of harmonious balance. (Fig. 3.2) The opposing qualities of *yin* and *yang* are viewed as interdependent and complementary. They create and control each other. When *yin* grows, *yang* declines, and vice versa.

The theory of *yin* and *yang* was well exposited by the time of Confucius in the fifth century B.C. In the West, we also accept the principle to a degree—male and female, hard and soft, good and bad, positive and negative electrical charges. It is proven by the law of charges that nothing in the physical world functions without positive and negative electrical charges. However, the perpetual interplay of *yin* and *yang* is the foundation of the Chinese (oriental) thinking and treatment of the body. Thus everything in life can be categorized according to its *yin* and *yang* components.

TARGET POINT

Yin and *yang* represent the perfect and harmonious balance of all elements of the universe according to Chinese methodology. *Yin* and *yang* are an integral part of Chinese medicine.

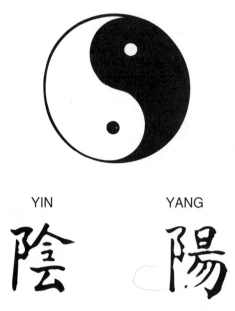

YIN   YANG

陰   陽

Fig. 3.2 The Chinese concept of the universe was based on the balance between *yin* and *yang*. Here are the Chinese characters for *yin* and *yang*, and the famous symbol.

YIN AND YANG

YIN	*YANG*
(−)	(+)
Earth	Heaven
Female	Male
Space	Time
Night	Day
Autumn/Winter	Spring/Summer
West/North	East/South
Interior	Exterior
Cold	Hot
Dark	Light
Water	Fire
Moon	Sun

YIN AND YANG IN THE BODY

YIN	YANG
(Zo) solid organs	(Fu) hollow organs
Store but don't transmit	Transmit but don't store
Liver	Gallbladder
Heart	Small intestine
Spleen (pancreas)	Stomach
Lung	Large intestine
Kidney	Bladder
Pericardium	Triple warmer
Blood	Energy
Shape, structure, weight	Active, warm, responsive
Lower parts (earth close)	Upper parts (heaven close)
Front inside body	Back outside body
Bones, internal organs	Skin, muscles
Spirit	Intelligence, will
Upward, inside meridian flow from earth	Downward, outside meridian flow from heaven
Meridian role to transform, store, distribute blood	Meridian role to process food, eliminate waste
Defense in long-term illness	Defense in early illness

Kei Raku

The *yin* and *yang* organs correspond to a charting or channeling system in the body that the Japanese call *Kei Raku*, or meridian system as we have previously referred to it. The term *Kei Raku* is used to define the Kei (horizontal) meridians and Raku (vertical) meridians. These meridians or pathways flow near the surface of the body in a manner some Western scientists believe to be related directly to the neurophysiological system. Others believe that this meridian system is an entirely different system flowing both directions in the body alongside the blood and lymph systems.

The physical existence of this system has been the subject of controversy from the beginning of modern medicine and is still scientifically unproven to the satisfaction of the Western medical community. For those who do accept the meridian system concept, the consensus would agree that it appears to be more sympathetic to the function and actions of the nervous system than anything else. For the sake of this book, we will lean toward the nervous system as the most closely related anatomical system. Nevertheless, it is believed that the meridian system flows and corresponds to all parts of the body.

TARGET POINT

Acupuncture and *Shiatsu* are based on a system of meridians or energy pathways that flow throughout the body. Most concentration lies in the primary twelve meridians and two controlling meridians.

Tsubo

Along the pathways of the system are points called *Tsubo* in Japanese. Other terms for these points include acupoint, pressure point, motor point, and trigger point. Essentially all refer to the same points strategically located along the system. There are believed to be perhaps as many as one thousand or more points in the body. *Shiatsu* concentrates primarily on the most superficial points, a system of around 365 points.

The theory behind the system is that if pressure (or needle insertion) is placed on one or more points along the meridian, a corresponding stimulation will take place in connecting parts or organs located on

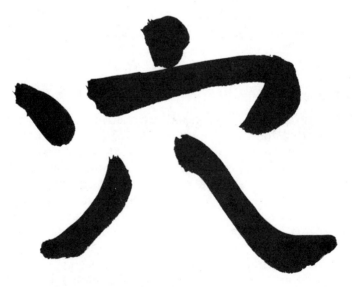

Chinese symbol for *Tsubo*. (Graphic by Lillian Sou.)

that same path. This would lend credence to the belief in the neurological similarity of reflex action. The *Tsubo* is not, of course, visible to the naked eye. Location of the *Tsubo* along any specific meridian varies from person to person and in accordance with the health and constitution of that person. The ability to locate surface *Tsubo* only comes with years of practical experience.

When doing acupuncture or performing *Shiatsu* from a healing standpoint, it's much more important to be accurate in order to achieve success in the healing. From a beauty and relaxation treatment standpoint, pinpoint accuracy isn't quite as critical and will be discussed more fully in a later chapter. In certain cases *Tsubo* can be pinpointed on the basis of a one to three location technique.

Location of *Tsubo*

1. Natural dent or hollow in the skin (e.g., temples): This is where the normal *Tsubo* energy is flowing properly and pressure applied is comfortable and easy to recognize by touch. Depth and duration of pressure is rather unlimited and not overly painful to the recipient.

2. Bump or nodule: This is where the *Tsubo* becomes blocked by a dysfunction along the pathway or tension. It feels like a bump and is quite sensitive to the touch, and due to the sensitivity can be painful to even slight pressure. Overt pressure or duration here will hurt the recipient and may cause reversal of desired result.

3. Assumption from charts: Following texts and charts allows the practitioner to proffer treatment even when not physically sure of the location of *Tsubo*. This is applicable in *Shiatsu* where the goal is purely preventative and for beauty purposes.

TARGET POINT

Tsubo are the acupoints located along the meridians that trigger corresponding responses along the meridian and related organs and systems. Acupuncture and *Shiatsu* pressure is exerted on these points to achieve the results of healing or general improvement of the structure.

With experience, the practitioner will develop sensory touch and will soon learn to locate *Tsubo* by touch. Touch is the best way to locate *Tsubo*, and this is why *Amma* massage in Japan traditionally has been performed by the blind. Where the visual senses have been lost the sense of touch has often been heightened. It is interesting to study *Shiatsu* with a blind person and to watch his/her acuity at locating *Tsubo*.

The *Tsubo*, as stated earlier, are located along a system of meridians. There are twelve primary meridians that are named in accordance with the corresponding *yin* or *yang* organs on which the pathways touch or cross. Most of the *Tsubo* used in acupuncture or *Shiatsu* are located along these twelve channels that flow near the surface of the body.

There are actually two more that run in the midline of the body and are considered important along with the twelve primary meridians. The extra two are called the governing vessel (GV) and conception vessel (CV) or directing vessel (DV). The original twelve are named for their six *yin* and *yang* organs. These are the ones we will remember. However, for the sake of reference, there are actually eight extra meridians, twelve muscle meridians, twelve divergent meridians, and fifteen connecting meridians all crisscrossing the body in different patterns. The number of *Tsubo* or acupoints along each meridian varies, but all the points on the meridian affect the organ after which they are named.

The names of the channels, the abbreviations for charting, and their relationship to *yin/yang* follow.

Meridians	Initials	*Yin/Yang* Reference
Lung	LU	*Yin*
Large Intestine	LI	*Yang*
Stomach	ST	*Yang*
Spleen	SP	*Yin*
Heart	H	*Yin*
Small Intestine	SI	*Yang*
Bladder	BL	*Yang*
Kidney	K	*Yin*
Pericardium	P	*Yin*
Triple Burner	TB	*Yang*
Gallbladder	GB	*Yang*
Liver	LIV	*Yin*

These two meridians govern all the others:

Governing Vessel	GV	*Yang*
Conception Vessel (also called Directing Vessel—DV)	CV	*Yin*

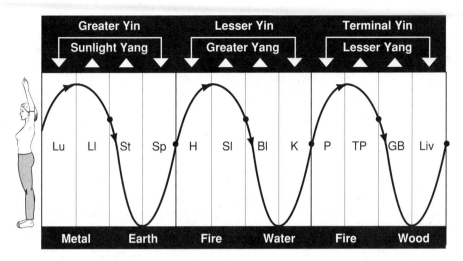

The movement of *Ki* through *yin* and *yang* channels.

Flow of Energy

It is interesting to note that the flow of energy throughout the entire *Ki* system follows a specific pattern. The *yin* and *yang* are specifically paired and complete a cycle in twenty-four hours. There is a peak activity time of two hours and a corresponding low time twelve hours later. This helps acupuncturists and physicians to base certain diagnoses on these phases. It is believed that the optimum time to treat the person is during the two-hour peak period. The cycle of energy begins with the lung meridian and flows in order through the liver meridian. The flow in the meridians follows three specific cycles. Each cycle contains four meridians.

TARGET POINT

The entire meridian system follows an organized and logical system of flow according to the *yin* and *yang* meridians.

In *yin* meridians, the energy flow is mainly upward from the feet to the chest and out to the fingertips. (Fig. 3.5) In the *yang* meridians, the energy flow is downward from the hands to the head and down to the feet. (Fig. 3.6) The meridian system is built anatomically to balance the function of all the body's mechanisms, circulatory, respiratory, digestive, reproductive, nervous, excretory, mental, and nutritional.

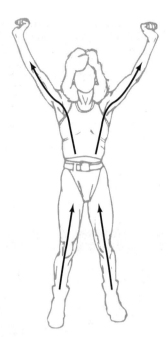

Fig. 3.5 *Yin* meridian. Energy flow is upward from the feet to the chest and out to the fingertips.

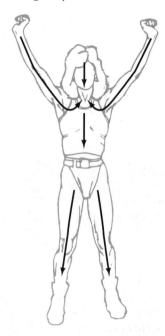

Fig. 3.6 *Yang* meridian. Energy flow is downward from the hands to the head and down to the feet.

THE FIVE ELEMENTS

In addition to the theory of *yin/yang* and the meridian system *(Kei Raku)*, another system was used to categorize most aspects of life, nature, and medicine. This was called the Five Elements, which also presented all aspects of life in a balanced format. The combination of *yin/yang* and the Five Elements formed a strong groundwork for understanding everything. The Chinese divided everything into one or several of these five categories. The five elements are: wood, fire, earth, metal, water.

Creating the Elements

Wood will burn to create a fire; the ashes left behind feed the earth; metal is mined from the earth; water condenses on cool metal; water feeds the wood to grow. (Fig. 3.7)

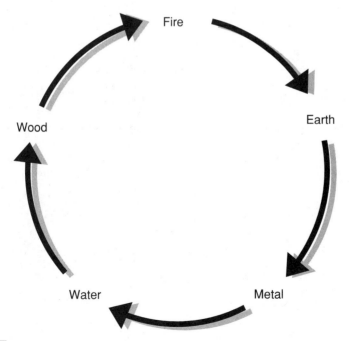

Fig. 3.7

Balancing the Elements

There is also a cross-referencing mechanism to keep the five elements in balance. Wood stabilizes the earth; the earth holds water; water controls fire; fire melts metal; metal (ax) cuts down wood. (Fig. 3.8)

When the Five Elements are used in conjunction with *yin* and *yang*, *Shiatsu* treatments can be much more effective. Certainly when a medical practitioner has the benefits of all these interrelated diagnostic tools to ascertain an illness or ailment, the results of acupuncture, *Shiatsu*, or any other healing practice is more effective. In the same way, we may choose to utilize some of these elements and characteristics to better understand the client we're treating.

TARGET POINT

The five elements of wood, fire, earth, metal, and water form another system to categorize all nature and, when included with *yin* and *yang*, form a creative system for analysis and diagnosis.

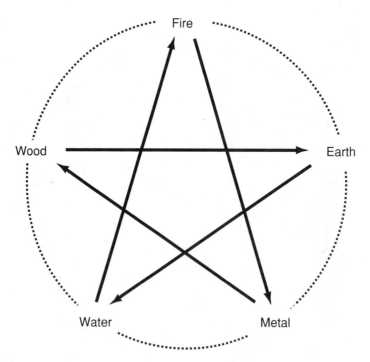

Fig. 3.8

The chart comprises information from a number of sources and is not conclusive to all students of Eastern medicine. However, this author hopes that the simplicity of the chart will assist the reader in a better understanding of the overall relationship of *yin/yang* and the Five Elements.

YIN/YANG AND THE FIVE ELEMENTS

Description	Wood	Fire	Earth	Metal	Water
Yin	liver	heart	spleen	lungs	kidneys
Yang	gallbladder	small intestines	stomach	large intestines	bladder
Direction	east	south	center	west	north
Season	spring	summer	transition	autumn	winter
Color	green	red	yellow	white	black
Sense	sight	words	taste	smell	hear
Emotion	anger	joy	worry	grief	fear
Flavor	sour	bitter	sweet	hot	salty
Spirit	mind soul	mind	intellect	body soul	will

FUNCTIONS OF SHIATSU

Acupuncture, as we all know, is the use of needles inserted into the *Tsubo* along a meridian to relieve pain or to correct a dysfunctional organ. Acupressure or *Shiatsu* can also be used in a healing and corrective capacity. The mechanism that causes the healing is not clearly known by Western methodology, but the effect of pressure on one part of the meridian has a relaxing or healing effect on another part.

In recent years it's also been interesting to learn that pressure applied on painful parts of the body can stimulate the opiate receptors in the brain and other tissues. This causes the natural production of or release of endorphins (endogenous morphine). Endorphins are considered to be five to ten times more powerful than morphine and when released are able to inhibit the transmission of pain signals through the spinal cord. *Shiatsu* pressure in tender areas may release endorphins to self-regulate pain, thus helping to restore the body to comfort and harmony. This functions in a similar way to the "runner's high" experienced by protracted periods of running.

Pain relief is certainly one of the most important functions of *Shiatsu*, even though estheticians and massage therapists are not officially doing *Shiatsu* for that purpose. In addition, *Shiatsu* has the ability to relax the body, stimulate the entire meridian system and increase energy, balance *yin* and *yang* for overall health, and relieve stress and fatigue.

TARGET POINT

Shiatsu helps to:

1. Self-regulate pain and discomfort through the natural release of endorphins.

2. Increase energy to the entire body.

3. Relax the body, relieve stress, reduce fatigue.

4. Through the concept of *yin/yang* balance, restore the overall well-being of the whole person by invigorating the skin, stimulating the various circulatory systems (blood and lymph), balancing the endocrine and digestive system, facilitating the normal functioning of the organs.

SHIATSU CLIENTS

According to Chinese and Japanese tradition all humans and their pets should receive *Shiatsu* treatments on a regular basis, whether localized for an area of discomfort or for the whole body to relieve fatigue. As you will learn in the practical application part of the book, *Shiatsu* can be done in facial treatments, body treatments, or in localized areas. Therefore, *Shiatsu* is valuable for all individuals.

In facial treatments, if *Shiatsu* is performed without any premassage, it is also very effective on recent postsurgical face-lifts and the like. The esthetician may also develop specific *Shiatsu* treatments for local areas, such as the eyes, for promotions, to be used in conjunction with a product or treatment, or just for variation. *Shiatsu* can be done in a full hour's treatment or as a mini treatment of fifteen to thirty minutes. This will be further broken down in the practical application chapters.

TARGET POINT

Shiatsu can be done on anyone, after surgery (carefully), over the entire body, or as a local spot treatment.

Contraindications

As with any treatment, I suggest you do not perform *Shiatsu* if there's any question about the health or applicability of the treatment. Caution must be taken when doing *Shiatsu* on anyone with a vascular problem such as hemophilia, diabetes (bruises easily), areas of telangiectasia (distended capillaries), and other systemic disease. Areas of inflammation and edema can be dangerous if the technician is not well trained, so if unsure these areas should be avoided along with areas of open lesions or infections. There are specific areas and times when it's best not to perform *Shiatsu* on a pregnant person. As you will learn in the practical section, the amount of pressure will also clearly be a determinant of contraindication of treatment.

TARGET POINT

Contraindications of *Shiatsu* are:

1. Vascular problems
2. Pregnancy (in certain areas)
3. Open lesions, areas of edema, infection, inflammation
4. Telangiectasia

SUMMARY

The Chinese system of *yin, yang,* meridians, and Five Elements all combine to provide the physician, esthetician, or massage therapist with a variety of tools to analyze and treat the whole person. Whether for healing or just for beauty and well-being, *Shiatsu* is unsurpassed as a therapeutic modality. Perhaps with more study and understanding, *Shiatsu* could easily become the foremost treatment modality in the armament of the esthetician or massage therapist as it is for some physicians who subscribe to both acupuncture and Western medicine.

Felix Mann from England stated in his book, *Acupuncture, The Ancient Chinese Art of Healing and How It Works Scientifically,* ". . . I tend to specialize in those diseases where Acupuncture is the better method of treatment; combining the Acupuncture with Western Physiology, Pathology, diagnostic methods, and if appropriate, ordinary drugs."

So the esthetician or massage therapist should approach *Shiatsu* in a manner in which both traditional massage and treatment may be used in conjunction with *Shiatsu* to achieve the optimum results physiologically and to relax and restore the client's whole being.

REVIEW QUESTIONS

1. What is *Ki*?

2. What was central to the understanding of the ancient Chinese philosophy, science, and culture?

3. Discuss some attributes of *yin* and *yang* overall.

4. What are some aspects of *yin* and *yang* in the body?

5. What are meridians? What is a *Tsubo* and where is it located?

6. How many meridians are normally considered in *Shiatsu* treatment?

7. What is the difference in the energy flow between *yin* and *yang*?

8. What are the Five Elements?

9. What are three results of *Shiatsu* treatment?

10. How can overall harmony be achieved?

CHAPTER 4

指圧

Benefits and Cultural Influences

CULTURAL INFLUENCES IN TREATING THE CLIENT

There are many differences in the cultural experiences of different parts of the world. We are all a product of our own local collective cultural experiences, but it is interesting to understand other cultures. When it comes to *Shiatsu*, it's particularly important to understand some of the differences in Eastern and Western concepts in health and beauty. We have certainly discussed it in great length in the historical development of *Shiatsu*, but from a practical standpoint we need to look at the concept of "touch" and how it becomes an important aspect of the utilization of *Shiatsu*.

Touching

Touch to a certain extent is a natural and instinctive reaction. Touching someone in different cultures takes place in different ways. In America, for example, shaking hands upon meeting someone is natural, proper, and expected. If you already know the person, perhaps a hug or kiss or both is in order. On the other hand, in most Eastern cultures, such as in the case of the Japanese, hugging and kissing is not a typical greeting. Bowing is much more the norm, not touching. The number and depth of the bows can often reflect the degree of respect. An interesting dichotomy takes place here, though. Although we hug and kiss even remote friends and acquaintances here, massage in general has been until recent years relegated to locker rooms and houses of ill repute.

Yet for the Oriental, massage, rubbing, and *Shiatsu* are a natural part of home life and take place between all members of a family from the youngest to the oldest. It's quite common for the younger generation to perform localized massages and *Shiatsu* on their elders. And going for *Shiatsu* or massage is commonplace. It's strange that our culture has held such disdain for such a beautiful, healthful practice when we readily hug and kiss.

As strange as this may appear to the student of *Shiatsu*, it's vital to understand later when it comes to marketing the *Shiatsu* service. You will have to teach the average consumer not only the physiological benefit of *Shiatsu*, but also the concept of getting the treatment in the first place. Current estimates guess that less than one-third of the entire American population have ever had a body massage, so it is logical to assume that less than 10 percent of those who have had massage have ever experienced a full body *Shiatsu* treatment. What a fantastic marketing opportunity.

TARGET POINT

Although Americans are a touching society from a greeting standpoint, estimates show that less than one-third of the population have ever had a body massage, much less *Shiatsu* massage, so the technician must clearly understand that to be successful he/she must educate the consumer about the need and value of *Shiatsu*.

Mind Body

Another important point that must be kept in mind when developing a program for *Shiatsu* treatments is the great history Eastern cultures have for total mind and body harmony as well as health by natural medicine. America has no such history, and holistic practitioners are often viewed as nuts or crackpots. This historical dependency on scientific medicine and incredible curative abilities related to modern medical science should not be discounted at all in the opinion of this author, whose life has been saved twice due to the tremendous success of American medicine.

But at the same time, there is room for more consideration of naturalism for health preservation and prevention of disease. It's well known now that the consumer trends lend themselves to holistic and alternative health practices. *Shiatsu* can be a wonderfully valuable tool for the beauty and allied health professional in health maintenance and relaxation of the human being.

TARGET POINT

Eastern medical precepts: Preserve health and prevent disease. Western medical precepts: Cure disease then restore broken health. Esthetician, massage therapist, beauty specialist: preserve good health, relax, restore and hopefully thereby prevent disease.

MENTAL/PHYSICAL RELAXATION

Relaxing and restoring the client is, of course, the very root of our treatment goal. As has been discussed to some degree in earlier chapters, relaxation has been proven scientifically to have restorative capabilities on the body. When we speak of relaxation, we must remember that there is mental and physical relaxation. When doing a *Shiatsu* treatment it is imperative that you relax not only the body but also the mind. The combination of mental and physical relaxation is a basic tenet of *Shiatsu*. The effect of the treatment is further enhanced if the technician is also completely relaxed physically and mentally. When treating a client, *Shiatsu* is not a modality to use in a rush.

When we speak in practical terms about what *Shiatsu* is going to do for the person receiving the treatment in a nonmedical setting, what are we talking about?

Stress and Fatigue

We are marketing to the client to do a number of things, the predominant one being the relief of stress and fatigue. Stress and fatigue are not the same. Fatigue is most often a result of stress or overexertion. Since stress causes fatigue and the person we treat today most often suffers from a lot of stress, then the stress-related fatigue will naturally be a large part of the potential client base. But even within the concept of fatigue, there are really two kinds.

Mental Fatigue

Exhaustion from emotional overload (high-stress job, the mother with triplets, etc.) or highly active mental work (the typical example being a person who works with numbers all day).

Physical Fatigue

Extreme under- or overexertion using the physical body. An example of underexertion-based fatigue is the person who's had the flu and been in bed for two or three days. Part of feeling bad is a lack of the normal level of movement and exercise. Overexertion can be demonstrated by the person living in Texas who decides to take a trip to Colorado for the first time in ten years to go skiing and spends the day on the slopes. Providing the person is not injured that day, the feeling of physical exhaustion at the "apres ski" is overweighed by the feeling of elation, until the next morning. And then the fatigue has really set in.

TARGET POINT

Do not overlook the importance of the two types of fatigue, mental and physical, because both can cause the metabolism not to work at optimum condition. *Shiatsu* can facilitate this process.

Metabolism

In a very simple way, let's briefly look at part of the cause of this exhaustion and how it affects the body. About 450 muscles in the body produce most of the movement. The contraction of the muscle to produce movement results from a complex process of metabolic activity that produces the energy. Indirectly the energy producing the muscle movement is generated by activities of the digestive process. When food is eaten, it begins digestion in the stomach, is then absorbed through the duodenum, and eventually passed to the liver where nutrients are converted to glycogen. Glycogen combines with oxygen from the lungs and is distributed through the body via the blood system, and some of the energy produced also causes the nerves to react and stimulate muscular activity.

At the same time, the neurological system reacts to input from the brain telling the nerves to generate muscular activity. For our purposes in *Shiatsu* and massage, the result of the metabolic process of digestion is very important because one of the byproducts of the metabolic process is a substance called lactic acid, which has a tendency to build up and is a major cause of fatigue. The entire subject of metabolism is very important and should be studied in great depth.

For the sake of this book, suffice it to say that metabolism is the entire life cycle, that is, the taking in of nutrients, utilization by the body of the important substances, and the elimination of the waste materials. Although in massage and *Shiatsu* we tend to show more interest in the elimination aspect because of the buildup of lactic acid in the body, it's also helpful to know what the client should be putting in the body as well.

TARGET POINT

Metabolism is important to understand and to be able to explain in simple terms to the client due to the tremendous effect *Shiatsu* has on its improvement. Metabolism is the intake of nutrients, utilization by the body of the important substances, and the elimination of the waste materials. The balance of both intake and elimination is indirectly enhanced by *Shiatsu*.

Lactic Acid Buildup

Why is lactic acid important to us? When there is a buildup of lactic acid, muscles tire more easily. This causes stiffness and soreness, can inhibit proper muscular function, and causes the lumps and bumps we so often find on the shoulders of our clients. *Shiatsu* can be used in this case to apply pressure directly over the areas of buildup to stimulate the overall circulation and metabolism, thereby helping the body to naturally rid itself of unneeded toxins and wastes. This process helps the body to do its own job better and results in increased energy in the whole person.

Mental fatigue and stress can, in likewise fashion, cause the body's system to be stressed, which results in interrupted metabolism also. When blood and lymph flow are not at peak performance, neurological response is affected, nutrition reaches the muscles more slowly, elimination of wastes and toxins is retarded, and the overall energy level of the person is reduced. The end result is still the same—fatigue, sore muscles, stiff shoulders, energy loss, sluggishness, all of which can be alleviated to some degree by *Shiatsu*.

TARGET POINT

Lactic acid buildup is a byproduct of ineffectual metabolism that the technician can often readily recognize by the lumps and bumps on the shoulders. Helping to disperse this waste material is a common result and benefit of *Shiatsu*.

Ambiance

As was briefly mentioned earlier, the other important part of the treatment itself is the atmosphere in which it is offered. In treating the typical American client, it should be kept in mind that the overall ambiance is tantamount to the success of the program. How can a client relax in a dirty, unpleasant environment where a technician might not have even changed the sheets from the last client? It wouldn't matter how technologically great the technician was in this situation. The client would, of course, be smart to refuse treatment, but if she didn't, would she really relax and receive its full potential benefit? No, of course not. Hopefully this never happens, but the point is to demonstrate the importance of ambiance as a treatment enhancer/facilitator.

Offering a Japanese ambiance is great so long as it doesn't go overboard. A well-known, highly respected cosmetic company in Japan attempted to launch their line in America many years ago and thought the launch would work most successfully if kimono-clad salesgirls did the promotions. The idea seemed great at first and certainly drew a lot of attention in department stores around America, but the sales didn't happen as they hoped and they lost millions of dollars. What they did not take into account was the fact that the American woman thought the kimono was beautiful and the launch interesting, but it did not give the impression that this cosmetic line would be appropriate for the American consumer. (As an aside, that cosmetic line relaunched again in America a few years later with an all-American campaign and has been doing well ever since.)

The point is, yes, it's great to offer a little of the oriental flair to the ambiance, but don't get carried away. In Japan at the Namikoshi Institute, clients are treated on thin pads on carpeted floors. This author doesn't really advocate you offer full body *Shiatsu* treatments on the floor, but it certainly doesn't require the traditional tatami mat in Japan either. The addition of slightly oriental music, if quiet, will add to the ambiance, and of course the product you choose to use in conjunction with the treatment may also add to the ambiance. Products will be discussed in a later chapter, but in traditional *Shiatsu* treatments, no products are used at all. The ambiance of the treatment can truly facilitate its effects.

SUMMARY

The value of *Shiatsu* from a purely beauty and health preservation standpoint should be obvious. Without playing doctor or attempting to cure a thing, massage and *Shiatsu* can go a long way just to relieve the symptoms mentioned and produce tremendous effects of well-being on the client. *Shiatsu* helps a person revive and refuel his or her own system. It guarantees a loyal and happy client. And the beauty of it all lies in the simple fact that *Shiatsu* is totally natural, completely holistic, and requires nothing but the talent and caring of the technician. And with the addition of the ambiance, music, and proper client handling, the value of *Shiatsu* is unsurpassed in the repertoire of the technician.

REVIEW QUESTIONS

1. What is an example of an interesting difference between the cultures of America and Japan?

2. How is massage (and *Shiatsu*) viewed in the American home versus the Japanese home?

3. What is metabolism?

4. What are the two types of physical fatigue?

5. What can lactic acid buildup cause?

6. How can *Shiatsu* help reduce lactic acid buildup?

7. Why is ambiance important in a *Shiatsu* treatment?

PART II

THE PERFORMANCE OF SHIATSU

CHAPTER 5

Effects of Shiatsu

Research has shown in numerous cases the impact touch has on the body, how some children grow up more stable because of the holding and nurturing of their mothers while still infants than children left in hospital nurseries. Research tells of certain animals who survive after birth only if the mother immediately licks off the baby. Animals that weren't licked off often died of some kind of internal functional failure. Hence, the impact of tactile stimulation may be a fundamental and essential ingredient of life that we have yet to fully understand. We do know that it seems to be a part of the healthy development of every kind of organism. It's also an interesting element of treatment for the client as well as the technician. Before going into the application of *Shiatsu* on the client, it's valuable to understand a little more about the impact touch has on the human body.

TOUCH

Without making this a text on the anatomy and physiology of the skin, it's useful to consider the skin and its relationship to *Shiatsu*, not only from the client's standpoint but from the technician's as well. As has been stated earlier, *Amma* massage in Japan was originally based upon the idea that a blind person was best suited to massage because of the superior refinement of the sense of touch. Touch is integral to the success of *Shiatsu* for both giver and receiver.

TARGET POINT

Perhaps the mechanisms of touch aren't fully understood yet, but we know that the tactile response to touch can give a baby a sense of safety or save an animal's life at birth. The sense of touch has resounding effects on the health and well-being of us all.

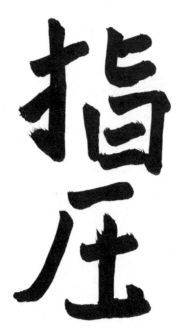

Chinese symbol for Shiatsu. SHI = finger, ATSU = pressure. (Graphic by Lillian Sou.)

The entire concept of *Shiatsu* is the idea of Shi (finger) and atsu (pressure), a massage therapy using pressure from the fingers and hands of the technician to the body of the recipient. Just the touch of the fingers to skin causes differing degrees of sensation. All sensations first sensed in the skin are transferred back to the brain for action by the nervous system. An organ this complex, as we have shown, deserves very careful handling. *Shiatsu* is, in the essence of it, quite simple to do once you are knowledgeable and experienced.

For the novice, however, it takes serious concentration and focus to perform the treatment to this highly sensitive tactile organ effectively, all the while developing a more sensitive sense of touch and point of reference. The important point for us to remember in order to master the art of *Shiatsu* is to be cognizant from the start of the inherent and dramatic effect touch has on your client, as well as you. It is, therefore, an art that takes focus, concentration, and practice to really be able to do well.

TARGET POINT

The trick to *Shiatsu* is to develop a sense of knowing where and how much pressure to apply in a treatment. Developing this sense comes with practice, focus, and dedication.

Consider for a moment how complex the largest organ of the body, the skin, is. According to *Milady's Standard Textbook for Professional Estheticians,* one square inch of skin contains:

- 65 hairs
- 95-100 sebaceous glands
- 78 yards of nerves
- 19 yards of blood vessels
- 650 sweat glands
- 9,500,000 cells
- 1,300 nerve endings to record pain
- 19,500 sensory cells at the ends of nerve fibers
- 78 sensory apparatuses for heat
- 13 sensory apparatuses for cold
- 160-165 pressure apparatuses for perception of tactile stimuli

There are sensory nerve fibers in the skin that react to four basic sensations: pressure, touch, temperature (heat and cold), and pain. The sensory aspect of the skin is what we deal with most in understanding how and where the technician is to use pressure to perform the treatment and also to understand the comfort and response levels of the client.

Sensory Receptors

Within the skin are different sensory receptors that record the different sensations, many of them named after the scientists who found them. There are:

1. Free nerve endings—pain receptors from the many branches of nerves.

2. Ruffini endings—notably heat receptors.

3. Pacinian corpuscles—encapsulated endings normally located between the dermis and subcutaneous layer that are receptors for deeper pressure.

4. Meissner's corpuscles—common receptors for light touch that are located in the dermis.

5. Krause's corpuscles—heat receptors located in the upper area of the dermis.

The previous relates to these receptors at skin level. In the deeper parts of the body, such as the muscles and joints, the roles may be different or overlap to a degree, and the additional Golgi tendon organ in muscle tendons responds to provide information on contraction, muscle stretch, and passive and active tension of the muscle. It's quite complicated if studied in detail, but the value in this brief review for *Shiatsu* is to understand that touch and different amounts of pressure will affect the system differently, changes in skin temperature will serve as a point of reference for the technician, etc. Also, as the technician's sense of touch becomes more refined the benefit and enjoyment of *Shiatsu* improves as well. It's exciting to realize that so many systems in the human body come into play during a *Shiatsu* treatment and that the human body can be re-energized by the effective application of differing degrees of touch on the various areas of the body.

TARGET POINT

There are four known receptors in the skin that relate directly to our sense of pressure, touch, temperature, and pain. For example, there are 1,300 nerve endings to record pain in an inch of skin.

Relief of Discomfort

The delicacy of touch is, of course, critical to the success of treatment, but touch to relieve discomfort is also a natural and instinctive reaction. When pain occurs suddenly, such as when you hit your funny bone, stub your toe, or cut yourself, applying immediate pressure to the area of pain is automatic and instinctive. Applying too much pressure or rubbing the area too hard increases the pain and discomfort, whereas the right amount of pressure decreases the pain.

The trick in *Shiatsu* is to learn how to properly and sensitively apply pressure and to learn how the body reacts in different areas and in different conditions. Understanding this aspect of *Shiatsu* is perhaps the hardest part of the learning curve, but it will come with time and dedication.

THE TECHNICIAN'S HANDS

Take a close look at the inside of your hands and study the contours of your fingers. You'll note an elevated tip on each finger and thumb. These elevated sections appear to have the greatest tactile sensitivity, and these pads lend themselves to effective *Shiatsu* treatment. Although the palms of the hands will also be used to perform *Shiatsu*, the primary tools of the trade will be the thumbs and fingers.

Contrary to many teachings, it is the opinion of this author that the tips of the fingers are never used for *Shiatsu*. The weight and pressure for application must emanate from the technician's body through the first pads of the thumbs and fingers. Pressure should also not be applied

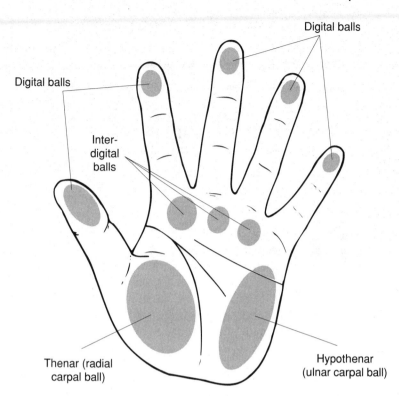

Digital balls

Digital balls

Inter-
digital
balls

Thenar (radial
carpal ball)

Hypothenar
(ulnar carpal ball)

at the point between the first and second joint of the thumbs or fingers. Using the tips or joints can radically change the quality and comfort of the client and can cause Carpel Tunnel Syndrome and other ailments rendering the technician useless in a few short years.

TARGET POINT

The elevated part of the pad of your fingers and thumbs are the most sensitive parts of your hands for use in *Shiatsu.* You must never use the very tips of the thumbs or fingers for applying pressure.

The majority of the pressure emanates from the position and movement of the technician's body. As much as possible, all pressure should come from the body. This not only balances and keeps the pressure more even from the client's standpoint but also takes the stress and strain off the hands of the technician. As you will see with practice, the use of the thumbs is predominant due to the stability and strength of its structure. There are several different positions of the hands and fingers available for use according to the area. The most common follow.

Proper Use of Hands and Fingers

Thumbs

Ideal for parts of the body where concentrated pressure is desired such as the temples, top of shoulders, along the spine, and center of calves. Thumbs can be used side by side, one at a time, or overlapped for greater pressure. When using thumbs, it's important to have the other four fingers spread to the side for added support. Sometimes the thumb and first or second finger are used together such as when doing the toes or fingers.

Fingers

You may choose to use just the first and middle finger, the first three fingers, all four fingers, or just one finger depending on the area. **Remember, use the first pad, not fingertips.** The index finger tends to have rather strong pressure and may be too strong on sensitive facial areas unless all fingers are used. The counterbalance of several fingers helps prevent too much pressure from just one. Sometimes greater pressure can be achieved when the middle finger overlaps the index finger. The choice of finger combinations will come naturally with practice.

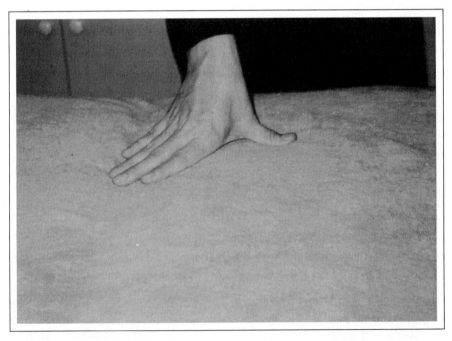

Thumb and finger positions when applying pressure with the thumb.

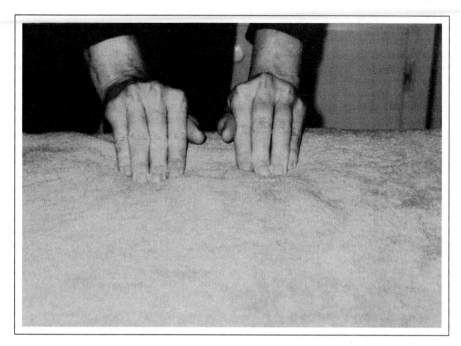

Four finger pressure.

Palms or Full Hands

(Often used on larger areas.) Full hands are used to cover the whole face at one time. Palms by themselves are helpful on the lower back and upper buttocks. Sometimes you will either use the inner palm (next to the thumb) or the outer palm (next to the little finger) for stronger concentration. When greater pressure is desired, hands may also overlap as with fingers. Overlapping palms also give a stabilizing effect on the back, shoulders, or head. Even though it would seem that overlapping hands or palms would make the pressure overly strong, with balance it often softens the pressure while adding depth. Full hands and palms are very useful in full body *Shiatsu* treatments.

TARGET POINT

Ideal pressure and control comes from applying pressure with your body, not your thumbs or fingers. Overlapping thumbs and fingers as well as overlapping palms sometimes increases the stability of the pressure force without being too strong if done properly.

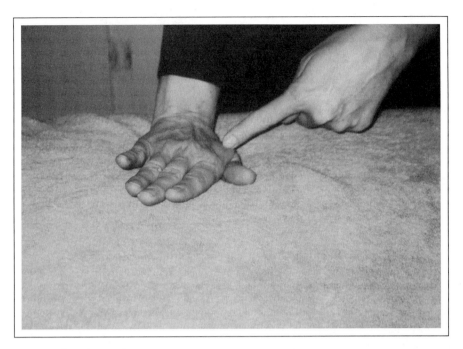

Inner palm pressure.

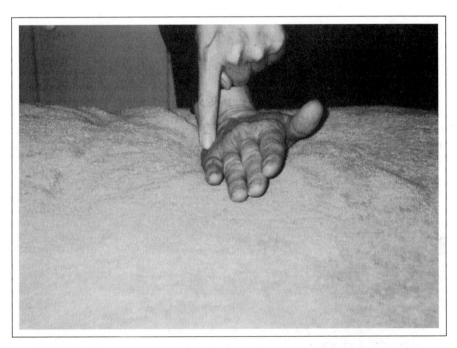

Outer palm pressure.

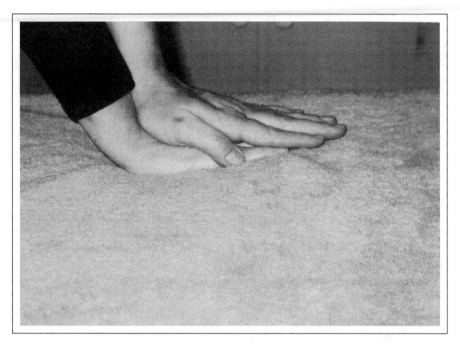

Overlapping palm pressure.

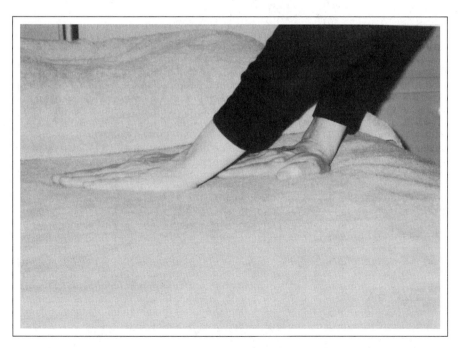

Pressure of full hands, side by side.

APPLICATION OF PRESSURE

CAUTION

UNDUE PAIN IS COUNTERPRODUCTIVE TO A GOOD TREATMENT.

The vital key to successful treatment is the ability to apply the correct amount of pressure to the area being treated. It should never be painful to the client. If the pressure exerted is so strong as to be painful, the application is incorrect.

There is, however, a fine line between pleasant discomfort and pain. It's difficult to describe the proper pressure because it varies widely from area to area and person to person. In reality, where there is acute pain, it may be indicative of a reflex or corresponding problem somewhere else along the meridian system or in a corresponding organ.

However, since we are not using *Shiatsu* to cure ailments, the mere fact that there is pain should only help us to understand better and then perhaps relieve that pain coincidentally while relaxing the area of discomfort. Remember, our goal is to relieve fatigue and stress and improve metabolism and circulation, so overly heavy pressure is not part of our treatment and completely unnecessary for the goal we have in mind. But if the discomfort is related to a buildup of lactic acid in the muscle or area, then it's very effective for relieving this condition and the discomfort is normal to a minor degree.

Heavier pressure may be used as long as the client is not hurting. "Comfortable pain" is the operative word. It is difficult to explain what's meant by comfortable pain. Flossing your teeth hurts a bit, but it feels good because you know you're getting the teeth clean. You want just enough pressure to know something is happening but not enough to cause pain. Also, sustained pressure for too long can cause the muscles to tense up and the opposite of our goal of relaxation can take place. Hence, mild pressure, for short amounts of time works best in esthetic treatments. If there is an area you feel you would like to concentrate on then apply pressure, move to another area, and come back again. It is strongly recommended that in addition to this book you obtain the videos and attend hands-on classes in order to really learn the movements, pressures to be applied, and rhythm.

TARGET POINT

Light pressure should be applied to sensitive or painful areas. Natural dents or comfortable *Tsubo* can handle more pressure. The amount of pressure should never be more than pleasantly uncomfortable.

Degree of Pressure

As previously stated, it's next to impossible to tell you how much pressure to apply because it varies for every individual and for the area being worked on. However the following will give you a simple frame of reference.

1. Light pressure may be calculated by reaching about two to three pounds of pressure on a weighing scale.

2. Medium pressure may be calculated by reaching about six to eight pounds of pressure on a weighing scale.

3. Heavier pressure may be calculated by reaching twelve to fourteen pounds of pressure on a weighing scale.

Depth and Duration of Pressure

At the beginning of a treatment, as pressure is applied to the first few areas, the client should be asked how the pressure is. If comfortable, proceed at the client's comfortable rate. It is prudent to ask periodically if the client is awake. If the client has gone to sleep, keep the pressure level about the same.

The duration of pressure also depends somewhat on the client, but normally most areas of the body should be pressed for approximately ten seconds per point. A particularly distressed area may require a little more or a little less. An excellent method for timing the length and depth of pressure is to inhale when you touch and slowly exhale as you apply the pressure. It is imperative in an effective *Shiatsu* treatment that you not rush. Slow, even, rhythmic movements are most effective. As you are first learning, it is wise to verbalize the following count exactly to develop good timing: Touch on 1, press on 2, release on 3.

Don't shorten the words, and say each line evenly. This will equate to approximately ten seconds, but you must do this out loud as you are practicing the pressure. Students in a practical class are required to count out loud for the first few days of classes until they get the hang of the timing. It's almost impossible to apply the correct amount of pressure for the right amount of time if you are trying to carry on a conversation. It's imperative that you quietly concentrate. Keep in mind also that you must try to balance the left and right hand pressure as closely as possible unless you're concentrating on a specific point.

TARGET POINT

Pressure should last about ten seconds per point and may be repeated in areas where more concentration is desired.

Pressure and *Tsubo* Location

As has been discussed previously, there are thought to be more than one thousand *Tsubo* or motor points in the body, but there are approximately 365 or so that we deal with directly in *Shiatsu*. Even at that you cannot possibly locate each point on every person. Additionally, even common *Tsubo* may be located in slightly different areas on each individual. This is why practice is the key to effective *Shiatsu* treatment. As we briefly discussed in chapter 3, the *Tsubo* may be located in different manners.

1. As a natural dent or hollow in the skin such as the temples or between the joints of the fingers. The common areas of dents normally indicate healthy energy flow and locating the point is relatively easy. These areas are not overly sensitive to average pressure.

2. As a lump or bump similar to the "golf balls" we often find when massaging someone's shoulders. These bumps may be indicative of lactic acid buildup or a blockage of the energy and even slight pressure may be quite uncomfortable. Light and repeated pressure is recommended here.

3. As shown on general anatomy charts or diagrams in this text. Since you are not learning *Shiatsu* for medical application, exact location of a specific *Tsubo* is not critical to the success of the overall area treatment. General application still increases circulation, improves metabolism and overall well-being, and relaxes.

The beginning student of *Shiatsu* will certainly have difficulty discerning dents and bumps, but it's exciting to develop better perception. A good practice is to just glide your thumbs or fingers up and down the arm feeling the lumpiness between the muscles. Another very lumpy area is the head, if you can find a bald person or someone with short light hair who will allow you to practice. Do not feel frustrated in the beginning; this will come naturally as you become more familiar with the practice.

TARGET POINT

Initially students will learn the location of most points by diagram or chart but with experience will develop the ability to sense most dents and bumps by touch. This will come naturally with experience.

Caution in Pressure

As has also been discussed, *Shiatsu* can be done on almost anyone, even after a recent face-lift where the skin shouldn't be rubbed or massaged, but the amount of pressure must be considered. There are very few contraindications to *Shiatsu* and common sense will normally advise you when not to do a treatment. But as a reminder, do not do *Shiatsu* on:

1. Areas of telangiectasia (varicose veins, couperose, distended capillaries, or any other vascular disorder).

2. Abdominal areas during pregnancy, disease, or discomfort.

3. Any disease where pressure could be a problem.

4. Areas of open wounds, lesions, inflammation, infection, edema.

5. Any situation you feel is questionable. (You should request a physician's release prior to performing a treatment.)

And finally, anytime there is question about the amount of pressure to be applied, just lighten the pressure to the touch level.

TARGET POINT

Never apply too much pressure to any areas of vascular problems such as varicose veins, couperose, and the like. When in question apply next to no pressure on areas of potential concern.

IMPORTANCE OF TECHNICIAN RELAXATION

Concentration is critical to develop the tactile sensory ability to locate *Tsubo*, but it's imperative that you, the technician, also be relaxed. If you are stressed or in a hurry, you will not only have more difficulty finding the *Tsubo* but you will also have great difficulty in balancing your rhythm and pressure. *Shiatsu* is not a therapy that can be done in a rush. If you relax and have the right atmosphere, perhaps some quiet soft music, you will easily learn to develop a smooth natural rhythm and will breathe correctly as you perform the pressure in each location. As a new student, you may also practice on your family members, a pet, or even your own arm or leg to develop the timing. Many expert *Shiatsu* technicians also study Yoga, relaxation, and meditation techniques, not from a spiritual or religious standpoint but in order to improve on the actual application of *Shiatsu* for the optimum results.

In addition to mental relaxation, it's also good for the technician to perform warm-up exercises for the thumbs, fingers, and hands to relax and limber up before doing treatments. The more relaxed your hands are, the easier it is to remember that all pressure should come from your body weight, not your hands. Tight, tense hands will fatigue easily and will also not be as good a tool for detection of sensory conditions.

SUMMARY

The actual application and performance of *Shiatsu* is not really difficult. In the same way a skater, diver, or football player practices his or her skills, the practice and development of *Shiatsu* comes with time and the desire to excel. Many people can skate a little, but an Olympic skater has mastered the art by practicing for hours and hours. Developing the ability to sense *Tsubo* and to know how much pressure is literally a matter of desire and focus. The art of *Shiatsu* is incredibly rewarding to the client even from the novice for, remember, touch is a natural and desired instinct. The important characteristic for the technician to develop is the desire to do a great job and offer effective treatments.

REVIEW QUESTIONS

1. Discuss some of the features of one inch of skin.
2. Is a good sense of touch important in *Shiatsu*? Why?
3. What are the primary parts of the body used by the technician to do *Shiatsu*?
4. How long should pressure be applied and how hard should it be?
5. List a few major contraindications to *Shiatsu*.
6. Why is it important for the technician to be relaxed when doing a *Shiatsu* treatment?

CHAPTER 6

指圧

Preparation and Handling of the Client

This is probably the most important chapter in any book on body work. For the esthetician, it's imperative to understand that the psychology of working on a client's body is entirely different than working on the face. When working on someone's face, the technician doesn't have to take into account modesty or shyness on the part of the customer since the only part of the body that's exposed to touching is the face, neck, and upper chest.

However, depending on how the client is prepared for a body treatment, part or all of the body may be exposed at some point during the treatment. Proper coverage and draping is critical to protect the client's modesty. It doesn't make any difference how good at the technical part of the treatment you are if the client is uncomfortable because he or she feels that part or all of his/her body is bared.

If the person is shy, as is often the case in America, proper handling is the single most important factor in achieving the physical results desired as well as keeping the client coming back. Poor draping alone could be the cause of client loss and you might never even know what went wrong. If because of poor handling the client doesn't come back, it could further injure your sense of confidence in thinking you did something technically wrong when it was merely a matter of incorrect handling. So, depending on the type of body treatment being done, handling and draping may be somewhat different. Since the topic of this book is *Shiatsu*, we'll concentrate on issues related to it.

TARGET POINT

Good client draping may make you or break you in your treatment success potential.

For the trained massage therapist, most of the rules of draping and client handling will be the same. For *Shiatsu* on the body, there may be a few variations but if you learned proper handling, this will come quite naturally and quickly.

ROOM PREPARATION

Room Ambiance

As discussed in chapter 4, the ambiance of the setting goes a long way in creating an effective treatment environment. The amount of money spent on ambiance is not as important as the aura created for the client. In America, clients are frequently hesitant to take off their clothes for a treatment and many months and years wind up passing before that client finally enters your treatment room. If the ambiance is right, the shyness factor and time may be shortened. A few quick rules for proper ambiance follow:

1. The room or area must be pristine and immaculately clean.

2. Sheets and towels must be clean, fresh looking, and not stained or have a massage oil odor. A number of products are available to remove oil stains and rancidity from sheets. This is imperative. The bed must be freshly made up to look as if the client coming in is the only one you've ever had or intend to have.

3. Absolute sanitation and hygiene is critical. All implements and surfaces must be kept clean and disinfected between clients. The room itself must look and feel crisply clean. Any hint of poor sanitation practice and your client retention is history!

4. Oils and other products must be kept clean and fresh looking. It's very easy for a working bottle of oil to look grotesque. This is a no-no. Change bottles regularly or prepare enough oil for each client. All products should be pleasantly displayed because this will help sell your retail items. (This subject will be discussed more fully in the marketing chapter.)

5. Choice of color for the room, sheets, and towels is purely up to you. I personally like colors and patterns, so I use brightly colored, patterned sheets and colorful plain towels in my salon. Very dark sheets are more prone to staining. If your clientele is male and female, you may either have two different color combinations or choose a unisex combination. Either approach is fine.

    I would also suggest that you purchase new sheets and towels long before they get too faded or raggedy looking. When the sheets and towels look uninviting, the client either prefers to move on or subconsciously judges you as "cheap." This is particularly important in upscale environments where the client pays a higher price than the norm for the service. When your sheets and towels reach the point where they look bad, donate them to a women's shelter, children's home, or even the local beauty school. You may have the possibility of a tax write-off, but even if you don't getting them physically out of the salon allows you (forces you) to obtain and maintain attractive ones.

6. Personal attire is perhaps the most important thing. Whatever you decide to wear as a uniform, be sure it's immaculate, crisp, and clean beyond doubt. A dirty, stained lab coat or working uniform entirely defeats the purpose of the image you're trying to portray. The lab coat itself is designed to send the message of professionalism to the potential client. If it is ugly, dirty, or wrinkled, what is the real message being sent?

Regular street clothes are no more recommended for the body therapist than the esthetician. When doing a body massage or *Shiatsu* treatment, some form of uniform helps show your professionalism and takes the "person factor" out. This also helps people get over shyness. Consider the difference you would feel if you went to a new doctor who came into the treatment room in jeans and a T-shirt rather than the usual white lab coat. There's automatically a certain level of safety and confidence when a doctor dresses as a doctor should. This is true for the beauty professional as well. The operative word here is professional.

Even though I prefer colorful sheets and towels, for personal attire I prefer either a lab coat or white pants and shirt. Sometimes it may get too warm to work on the body in a lab coat so if you're wearing a white T-shirt and pants be sure that they look great, not like an old T-shirt you'd wear at home to clean house. If possible the shirt or pants should have a logo or some designation that advertises the salon, so it really looks like a uniform.

If you are prone to perspiring while you work, have two or three uniforms available to change into from time to time during the day. If your *Shiatsu* treatments are to be done in conjunction with massage, mud, or other possible staining treatments, again be sure to have extra uniforms around. After you've become stained with mud or oil, you can't just tell the client that you're sorry. How would the doctor look to you if he or she showed up in your treatment room with blood all over his or her lab coat?

7. It's important to have a clock on the wall for the technician to refer to during treatment for proper time control.

8. Music is always a great additive to the ambiance. Slightly oriental tones to the music may be very pleasant and heighten the marketability of the *Shiatsu* treatment. Do not get into the old historical Enka-type Japanese music. It's too "country westernish" for this sort of treatment. A very well-known musician such as Kitaro has great music for *Shiatsu*. Kitaro and similar music is available in large music stores or new age book stores. Other sources of interesting music are the new natural science, earth friendly, and bird sundries stores. When looking into environmental music, be cautious of music that has too many water sounds as they often force your client to need to go to the bathroom in the midst of treatment, which is time consuming and distracting for both you and the client. Music may be necessary to help soundproof the room from outside salon noises. Be sure the area can be kept quiet.

9. Lighting is another important issue for the room. Whenever possible, have the room lighting on dimmer switches that are near the technician so that depending on the stage of the treatment the technician can turn the lights up or down as desired. Wall sconces with upturned or indirect lighting are great. The room should be well lit for opening discussions, analysis, or consultation, but once the treatment begins, lighting should be low and subdued. This adds to the feeling of relaxation for the client.

TARGET POINT

Be very pristine and clean about all details related to the room. A clean operation speaks well for your professionalism. You will set yourself above the average salon by being sanitary and paying close attention to proper disinfection.

CLIENT CONSULTATION CHART

Just about the most important aspect of client care is proper documentation and charting. Everyone has their own idea of the perfect client consultation chart. Many choose to create their own whereas others prefer to purchase ones that have already been developed for sale by esthetic companies. The charts are important to have for several reasons.

1. A good client history gives you valuable information on the health and lifestyle of the client in order to perform better treatments.

2. Charting specific skin lesions or noticeable problems might protect the salon in the future against a potential erroneous claim from the client.

3. It's impossible for the busy salon and technician to remember all treatments, details about the client's personal life, or what was recommended for home usage. Good record keeping will refresh the technician's memory when the client returns.

4. Keeping good records of treatments and home care products allows for creative marketing on an ongoing basis for products and services the client hasn't tried.

Vital Information to be Included on the Chart

The style may vary in size and detail, but some items should always be on the chart. Important information includes:

1. Basic client information: name, address, phone numbers, physician phone numbers, date of birth if possible.

2. Medical history of diseases, disorders, medications, and allergies to medications and cosmetics.

3. Some lifestyle information: hobbies, business, time available for personal care, reason for visiting salon, cosmetics used, skin care areas of concern.

4. Section for technician analysis: skin type and conditions, areas of concentration, recommended programs, products and samples, personal things the technician wants to remember about the client, space for comments.

Along with the main chart should be home care recommendation pads where products can be recommended with usage and details. A copy should be kept by the salon and one given to the client.

The most important aspect of charting and record keeping is keeping the chart up-to-date and continuing to work off it. Filling a chart out and then ignoring it renders it next to useless. A computer system that holds and tracks all information is great, but most smaller salons do not have the really sophisticated tracking systems. So it is up to the salon owner and technician to be sure it's kept up-to-date.

Client charts should be kept in a filing cabinet or some secure place. Determination of salon ownership of these charts is imperative and the employee must know this. Charts must remain the property of the owner.

If the technician is leasing space in a salon, the technician owns the charts. If the technician is an employee, the salon owns the charts. In the event of termination of employment, charts must remain with the owner. Technicians will likely copy the information to move on, but keep in mind that the legal owner is the salon.

TARGET POINT

Client consultation charts are important for legal protection as well as proper client tracking. Good tracking will help the salon market new products and services within the existing clientele much more effectively.

MASSAGE TABLE SETUP

The sheets, towels, and blankets must be clean for each client. The blanket itself doesn't necessarily have to be washed between each client as long as the client's body hasn't come in direct contact with it or oil hasn't bled through the sheet. It's advisable to make a sheet cover for your blankets so that nothing touches them and wash the covers once or more a day as needed. The sheets and towels must be washed after each client. Some technicians just flip the sheet over and turn it around between two clients. This is not acceptable.

The table should be set up with client comfort in mind. Most massage tables today are well padded and have face cradles with holes for the client to breathe through when lying on the stomach. If padding is needed, you may choose to buy those egg-crate pads that you see often in hospitals. Blankets can be put on the table and then the sheets and towels over that for extra padding. After a blanket, sheet, and big body towel (bath towel is okay but bath sheets are much larger and cover the client better) have been put on the table or bed, a cover bath sheet or sheet and blanket should be placed on the bed for the client to be covered with.

Do not worry about using too many towels. Body treatments always require more towels than facial treatments because it's imperative that the client be well covered and kept warm. The bed should look smooth and inviting to the client upon entering the room.

It's good to have roll bolster pillows to put under the client's knees while he/she is lying on the back and a neck pillow for the back of the neck if necessary. Be sure the pillows are also covered and changed between clients.

WORK TABLE SETUP

Put a small towel on the counter or trolley before placing work products on it. This gives the client a very pleasant and clean impression. Set out the products you plan to use on the towel in the order in which you plan to use them. Normally in *Shiatsu* you will only need a proper hand sanitizer, massage oil, and powder for the treatment. Place another small towel nearby for drying your hands. Any bowls, sponges, shammies, or other implements you'll need for treatment should be placed on the work area towel before treatment begins. The most important aspect of this is to keep the table neat looking. Don't get messy or cluttered; this can give the client a very bad impression at the start.

> ### TARGET POINT
>
> The table and area setup should look as if the client about to enter is the first and only client ever to lie on those sheets. Color may be used effectively for mood and a pleasant environment but white is also very clean and professional.

CHOOSING PRODUCTS FOR TREATMENT

As has been stated previously, true Japanese-style *Shiatsu* requires no product application or clothing removal. However, it's recommended that *Shiatsu* in America be done directly on the skin after a short effleurage massage. Choosing the massage product is very important because of the danger of too much slip and scratching the client or slipping off the *Tsubo*.

Choice of Oil

The oil of choice must be a very light "dry" oil. Dry in this case means an oil that practically disappears, that is not greasy or too slippery. The novice may have to test a number of oils before clearly understanding the type of oil that is ideal for treatment. If you use a specialty oil designed specifically for *Shiatsu* you will be assured of the right texture. Experimenting will eventually teach you the texture of the oil you want. You can search for an oil that promises not to stain sheets. There are some that claim not to stain, but you should test this out for yourself as that's a difficult claim to back up. From an ambiance standpoint, a slightly oriental mood to the oil helps the treatment as well. This is a marketing issue more than a treatment issue, but hints of oriental notes are good— essences of jasmine, ylang-ylang, or lavender.

Choice of Powder

Some technicians prefer to do a light effleurage massage to open with powder and then do *Shiatsu* directly over that. Using powder is fine so long as you remember that it can make the skin dry. If your client already has dry skin, this is not recommended. Powder is often best used at the end of the treatment for finishing and polishing. I prefer to use oil and then finish with a powder to make the skin shine and to absorb any excess oil. This is particularly important on the feet between the toes and the hands between the fingers.

Choosing powder is similar to choosing oil. You want a smooth, soft powder that glides well but that isn't too drying. Talcum powder alone can be very drying. Corn starch-based powders are not quite as drying to the skin but are often rougher in texture. Fragranced powders are often shunned by the client so be careful in choosing perfumed powders that aren't specially made for the purpose.

Choice of Hand Sanitizers/Disinfection Procedures

Different states now have different requirements for sanitization, so be sure to check with your licensing authorities. You should use the proper legal sanitization products, but whatever you use be sure to use it after washing your hands just before beginning the treatment. Also, if your client didn't shower before entering the room for treatment (if you don't have a shower or there's no time for the shower), you'll at least want to sanitize the hands and feet of the client too as you begin to work on that area. But when sanitizing the client's feet or hands, be low key; you don't want the client to think that you think they have a disease. Do not, however, be low key about letting the client be aware that you sanitize your hands before treatment.

If you happen to have a nick or cut on your hands, be sure to wear gloves. If you are thinking that you can't do a massage or *Shiatsu* with gloves on, you're entirely wrong. You must practice with gloves because the truth is that you can easily feel and sense the skin even through them. Be sure they fit your hands well. There is a good chance that someday we will all be required to wear gloves for all treatments so you might as well get used to the idea. Wearing gloves protects both you and the client. If the client has a cut or lesion, again you should wear gloves.

The technician's fingernails must be immaculate and short. They must not protrude past the nail bed because of risk of cutting the client while applying pressure. Technicians who attempt to do *Shiatsu* with long nails not only risk injuring the client but also tell the experienced client that they don't care to be professional. Any experienced person will judge you immediately by the length of your nails. Estheticians know that long red nails are unprofessional in facial treatments, but it's even more critical in *Shiatsu*. If you think you can cheat in certain areas and use your fingers sideways, you again exhibit a lack of professionalism and the experienced client will soon go elsewhere.

TARGET POINT

Choose products carefully for your desired results, for ambiance, for convenience according to the treatment. There are a myriad of oils from which to choose. Choose oils that aren't too slippery or tacky. Powders that aren't too drying may also be used but are recommended for finishing purposes. Above all, the technicians's fingernails must be kept short to keep from injuring the client.

TREATMENT TIMING/CLIENT HANDLING

Timing for any treatment begins and ends within the time frame quoted on the menu. If a full body *Shiatsu* treatment is programmed for one hour that means exactly that—one hour from arrival in the room to departure from it. Full body *Shiatsu* treatments are normally one hour long. The treatment per area opens and closes with effleurage, with the bulk of the concentration on *Shiatsu* of course. If doing a full body, the front side of the body takes approximately thirty-five minutes and the back side approximately twenty-five minutes. When offering *Shiatsu* as an incremental treatment or for specific parts of the body, timing will be explained within the treatment chapters of this book. However, whenever timing is considered, remember that timing always means from arrival to departure.

As far as bookings on the master appointment book are concerned, allow ten to fifteen minutes between clients for selling time and clean up. It is also recommended to book an hour and a half for the first time a client receives a treatment to allow for full attention to the client without feeling rushed to get ready for the next one and to properly take care of the client's needs.

If possible, have a separate changing area away from the treatment room. Sometimes this is impossible in a small salon, but the problem with having the client change clothes in the actual treatment room is the time lost in waiting. And if the client intends to fix herself up and apply makeup she could tie up your room for a half-hour or more and this will hurt your business. You must be able to turn the room around quickly and move on into the next treatment.

On first time visits, have the client arrive fifteen minutes early to fill out your client history chart. Whatever chart format you have in mind is fine, but be sure to have one. When doing facial work, knowing a client's medical and lifestyle history is important to proper analyzation and sales followup, but it's vitally important in body work. As stated, the full body requires more attention to health histories, contraindications, etc. You need this information and there's nothing wrong with having the client arrive early. Then you want to take a few moments to review the chart before initiating the conversation and treatment.

After the treatment, have the client become fully awake and restored before having the final sales discussion and letting the person leave the salon. A good idea is to get the client up and offer a glass of water or juice while discussing the home care routine you want followed. Remember that even if the client comes to you strictly for *Shiatsu* it's an important opportunity for you to sell home care products for the body. This balances the treatment, improves the client's skin and well-being, and keeps the client locked to the salon.

TARGET POINT

Wise use of timing will make or break your business. When a treatment is scheduled for one hour, that means from arrival to departure. A first time client should be booked for one and a half hours to have plenty of time for charting, client consultation, treatment, and final home care sales.

SUMMARY

In a nutshell what this chapter is all about is presenting you, your salon, and your client to a professional, relaxed, and comfortable environment all the way around. Both you and your salon should be so clean that there is no room for doubt in the client's mind of personal health safety. The professionalism in room and setup adds credence to the treatment and enhances the enjoyment for the client. All that's left is a great treatment to ensure that you stand hands and feet above your competition. So much of what's been covered in this chapter is common sense for all beauty professionals, from the hairdresser to the esthetician or massage therapist. The sad part is to know how few pay attention out there in the salon world. If you pay attention to this, you're halfway to success, and believe it or not the sophisticated client knows it. Remember, your *Shiatsu* client is usually going to be sophisticated. You will mirror the level of your client by your professionalism.

REVIEW QUESTIONS

1. What is the most important factor in client draping?

2. Why is the client consultation chart so important?

3. How should the massage table and work area be set up?

4. What kind of lighting and music should be used in a *Shiatsu* treatment?

5. Why is cleanliness and sanitation so important in treatment?

6. What kind of massage oil should be used in *Shiatsu*?

7. Does it matter if the technician has fingernails?

8. What aspects of booking clients for treatment are important?

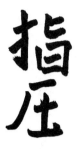

CHAPTER 7

Shiatsu for the Head, Neck, Chest, and Shoulders

In this and the next chapter, you will learn a variety of treatments using *Shiatsu*. There are a number of important points to keep in mind.

1. Since we are using *Shiatsu* for beauty and relaxation purposes, not medical or curative whatsoever, the precise order in which you choose to do each point doesn't matter. If at first you forget a specific area, don't worry. Just keep going. Each time you perform *Shiatsu* you will get better and better. Soon, the logical order and degree of pressure will come naturally to you. As discussed earlier, it is still advisable to take a practical course in *Shiatsu* to learn rhythm, balance, and depths of pressure.

2. True oriental *Shiatsu* doesn't require the removal of clothes or makeup or the use of massage oil. If you choose to do *Shiatsu* the more traditional way, it's advisable to have the client wear soft and loose clothing to facilitate your sense of touch in locating the *Tsubo*. In most treatments for the American market, however, I recommend the use of massage oils and removal of clothes and makeup. Please refer to chapter 6 for oils, setup, etc.

3. Always pay attention to the client chart and contraindications and discuss the amount of pressure with the client as you begin treatment and become accustomed to that particular person.

4. *Shiatsu* can be done alone or in conjunction with the traditional classical European massage movements. It can also be incorporated into aromatherapy and other treatment modalities. It is strongly recommended that effleurage (light, gentle stroking movements) be done just prior to *Shiatsu* and then immediately after. In other words, open and close the *Shiatsu* treatment with effleurage. Please use your own effleurage techniques or refer to *Milady's Standard Textbook for Professional Estheticians*, chapter 14. This chapter will

also give you some hand exercises to relax your hands and make them more limber for the *Shiatsu* treatment.

5. *Shiatsu* effects are heightened by your expert knowledge of the body's anatomy and muscular structure. You may refer to various anatomy books for a review of the muscular structure. For facial treatment, you may also refer to chapter 14 of *Milady's Standard Textbook for Professional Estheticians.*

TARGET POINT

Shiatsu, when used for beauty enhancement purposes, does not have to be done in any specific order. There is a logical movement from one point to the next when done in a pattern, but this will come easily with practice and experience.

SHIATSU TREATMENTS

Head and Scalp

Purpose

1. Stimulates circulation and subsequent nutrition to the scalp and hair roots, which promotes good healthy hair growth

2. Relieves stress and tension

3. Relaxes hair follicles allowing better absorption of conditioning agents

4. Helps stimulate sebaceous gland production to lubricate dry hair and improve the condition

Technique

Depending on whether a little *Shiatsu* is being done in conjunction with a shampoo or normal treatment, the technique may be broadened by using the entire inside of the thumbs around the curve of the index finger in a clamp-like full hand grip of the sides of the head and working back to the base of the head. If, however, the treatment is being done as a chargeable *Shiatsu* service, it's advisable to overlap the thumbs and work the entire head with the thumbs until you reach the base. The entire head will be lifted by the four fingers while pressing on the occipital area.

The treatment can be done on a wet or dry head at the shampoo area or at the hairdresser's station. Before beginning the *Shiatsu* be sure to massage the entire head with fingertips to open the treatment.

1. Press the main *Tsubo* at the crown of the head three times.

2. Move to the front of the forehead at the hairline. Apply pressure to three points about one-half inch apart from the center line to the top of the ear on the left side and then the right.

3. Move back about one-half inch to the next row of *Tsubo* and repeat left, then right. Repeat row after row until you reach the main crown point. On most heads you will have five rows from the forehead to the crown.

4. Depending on the position of the client, you may need to use one hand to brace the head from the forehead while using the other thumb and your body weight to press in toward the face on the back side of the head in the same manner, three points on each side of the center line left side, then right. Each row should also be about one-half inch apart. You should have about five rows from the crown to the base of the head.

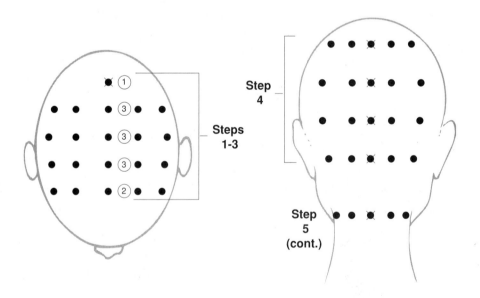

Location of pressure points, step by step.

5. The last row for the base of the head should be just under the occipital. Place all four fingers cradling the head, and this time your pressure should be applied with a lifting movement as if you would lift the head off the neck.

6. Apply pressure with thumbs to the temples.

7. Using the four finger and thumb vice-grip technique, apply pressure in three straight rows down the neck to the shoulders. The first time the four fingers of the right hand will be on the right-hand side of the neck. The second time switch hands and the four fingers of the left hand will be on the left-hand side of the neck.

8. Massage upper shoulders and apply pressure to *Tsubo* on the upper area of the shoulders as desired. Normally apply pressure to about three points on top of shoulder.

   End the *Shiatsu* treatment with relaxing massage of the entire head, neck, and shoulders. Proceed with scheduled treatment. Treatment may include a scalp mask, conditioning treatment, or normal chemical or styling work.

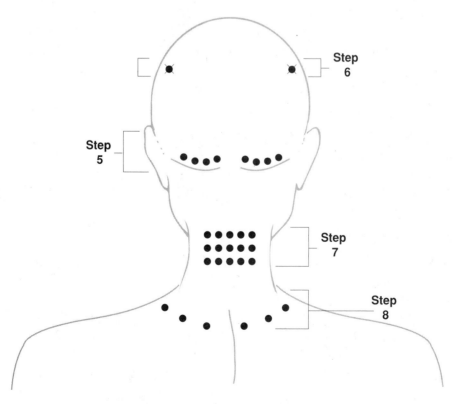

TARGET POINT
Shiatsu for the scalp is a great add-on service for the hairdresser and relaxes the client while improving the condition of the scalp and hair.

Full Facial Shiatsu

Purpose

1. Stimulates circulation without moving skin. If done without pre-massage, may be useful to stimulate natural healing for post-facial cosmetic surgical procedure (face-lift).

2. Relaxes the facial features thus reducing fatigue.

3. Increases nutritional exchanges and enhances absorption of products.

4. Relieves stress.

5. Relaxes facial muscles and also enhances subsequent treatment product absorption.

6. Helps even out skin tones.

7. Feels great and relaxes.

8. Indirectly improves all functions of the skin and body in the area treated.

9. Pressure around the eyes relieves fatigue, dryness, redness, and itchiness.

10. Pressure on the temples relieves stress and may help relieve tension.

11. Pressure in the sinus group will relieve pressure buildup, assist in decongesting the sinuses, and relieve pressure to the eye and forehead areas.

12. Pressure around the mouth helps freshen breath and brings nutrition to the mouth.

13. Pressure on the cheeks relieves stress and tension and relaxes the face, particularly for someone who talks a lot.

Technique

Warm up with relaxing effleurage for the entire face, neck, chest, and shoulders. Whether the full facial *Shiatsu* is being done as a quick part of the regular facial or as a specific service will determine your time allotment. If doing only as part of a regular treatment, you will have about ten minutes for the entire face as part of the massage. If so, apply light pressure only once to any area.

If doing as part of a special treatment (chargeable), the ideal is to apply pressure on stressed areas more and then do each section of the face from one to three times. (*Section of the face* refers to the charted groupings such as the forehead group, the eye group, and the mouth group.) Although the face may be done with different fingers and thumbs as well as with the full hands depending on the size of the face and technicians hands, the following may be helpful in determining which parts of the hands are normally used: We'll use thumbs for temples, three

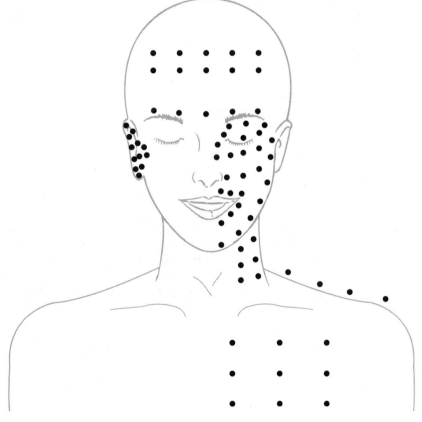

Full face, neck, and chest, with pressure points.

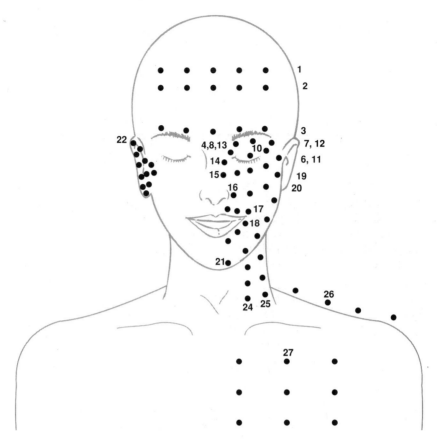

Pressure points, step by step.

to four fingers for facial points where face size and hands fit, and full hands and palms over eyes in full face movement.

Consider the face, neck, and chest divided into sections with about three rows within each section (some clients will have only two rows and some will have four). Movements are normally done from the center of the face or body outward and from the top of the head downward. Both sides of the face and chest will be done simultaneously so even, balanced pressure is required.

1. Using the first four fingers, start applying pressure at the upper row right at the hairline. (Fig. 7.5) Do three rows from the center of the forehead out to the top of the ears. Use middle and ring fingers or thumbs to apply pressure to the temples. (Fig. 7.6)

2. Slide to about the middle of the forehead and repeat with three rows out to the top of the ear. Repeat temples as desired.

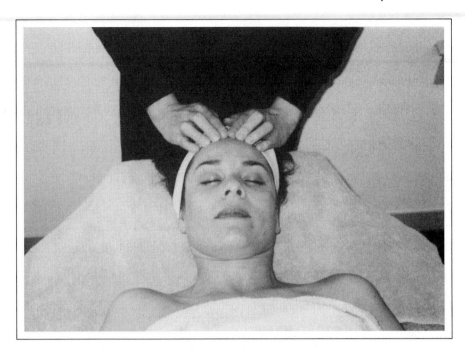

Fig. 7.5 Apply pressure at the hairline.

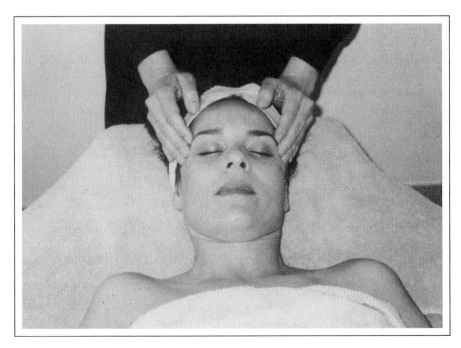

Fig. 7.6 Apply pressure to the temples.

3. The last forehead row should be right on top of the eyebrows. Repeat three rows. Repeat temples as desired.

4. Apply pressure with middle or ring finger to upper inner corner of eye just inside and under ocular bone. (Fig. 7.7)

5. Move to middle of upper eye; repeat pressure with same finger. (Fig. 7.8)

6. Move to outer corner of eye at junction of upper and lower eyelid; repeat pressure with same finger. (Fig. 7.9)

7. Apply pressure to temples with fingers or thumbs. (Fig. 7.10)

8. Repeat upper inner corner eye point.

9. Move to lower inner corner of eye at tear duct; apply lighter pressure with finger.

10. Move to lower middle of eye; apply light pressure with same finger.

11. Move to outer corner of eye (same location as outer corner when doing upper eye); apply pressure.

12. Repeat temples.

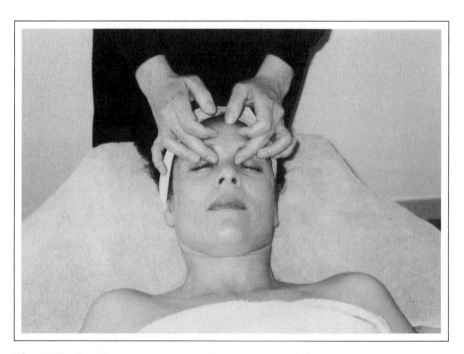

Fig. 7.7 Apply pressure to the inner corner of the eye.

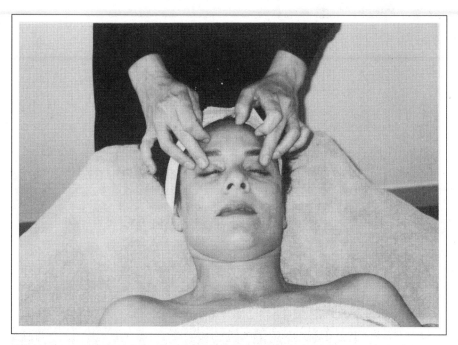

Fig. 7.8 Apply pressure to the middle of the eye.

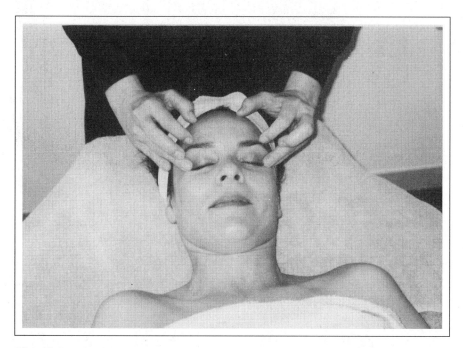

Fig. 7.9 Move to the outer corner of the eye and apply pressure.

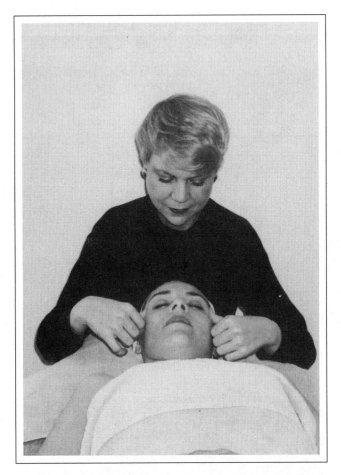

Fig. 7.10 Apply pressure at the temples, using the thumbs.

13. Repeat upper inner corner of eye.

14. Move to upper sinus area just below tear duct. Apply pressure with same finger. (Fig. 7.11)

15. Move slightly down and out to main sinus *Tsubo* and apply pressure. (Fig. 7.12)

16. Move to just under nostrils (deep dent) and apply pressure without blocking nostrils or applying pressure in toward nostrils.
    (Note: All three points for sinus are to be done on the face, not in or on nose itself.)

17. The upper lip area is to be done in a slightly lifting movement to be sure that pressure is applied directly to the gums, not the teeth.

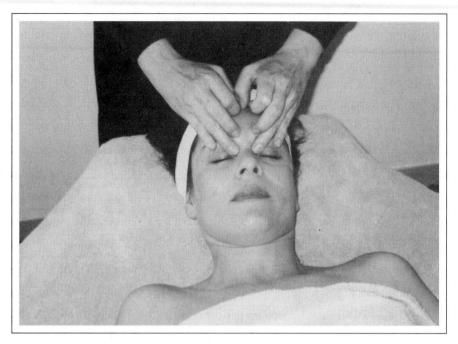

Fig. 7.11 Move to the upper sinus area and apply pressure.

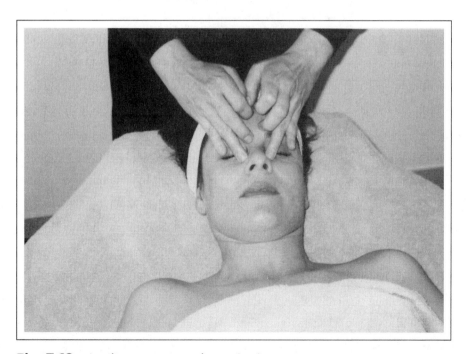

Fig. 7.12 Apply pressure to the main sinus area.

Four fingers may be used to apply direct pressure. If the area is small or the technician's fingers appear to be too large, apply pressure with the sides of the middle or ring fingers covering the entire upper lip area. (Fig. 7.13)

18. The lower lip area should be done in the same manner, either with direct finger pressure or sides of fingers in a slightly downward pressure to be sure the pressure is on the gums.

19. Move back up to the middle sinus point for finger placement reference. Using three or four fingers, apply pressure in three rows from that point directly on the cheeks out to the top of the ear. (Fig. 7.14)

20. Move down to the last sinus point under the nostrils to begin the middle cheek row. This row requires that the fingers lift up under the quadratus and masseter muscles in three rows out to the middle flap of the ear.

21. The last row will be done with four fingers starting on top of the center of the chin working out in three rows to the base of the ears. (Fig. 7.15)

22. The ear group will be done in two rows, one on the outer cartilage of the ear and the second on the inner heavier cartilage of the ear.

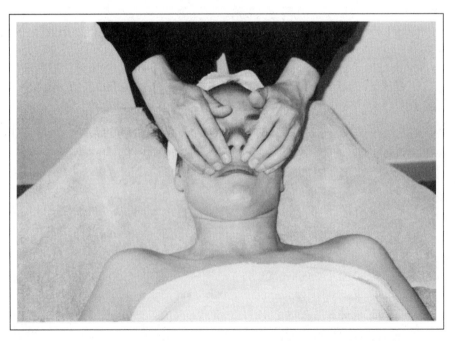

Fig. 7.13 Use fingers to apply pressure to the entire upper lip area.

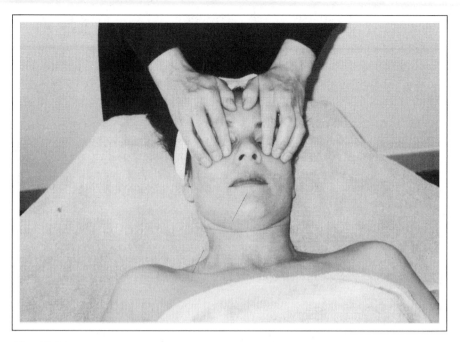

Fig. 7.14 Apply pressure in three rows from that point directly on cheeks out to the top of the ears.

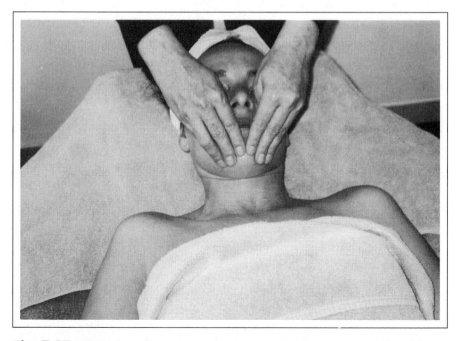

Fig. 7.15 Using four fingers, apply pressure to the center of the chin.

There will be approximately eight points very close together moving from the earlobe up and around to the top of the ear and then the ear flap. Pressure will be applied with thumb and first finger up and around with equal pressure on both sides. (Fig 7.16) The inner row will be with pressure mostly from the thumbs only while the fingers support the ears.

23. Apply full two hands pressure for the entire face. Placement of hands are flat on the face facing downward with the pads of the palms resting on the eyebrows. Hands do not cover the nose. Apply full even hand pressure and then open hands as if opening a book. Close hands and repeat pressure and opening technique three times.

24. The front sides of the neck are optional. Pressure is applied just next to the esophagus on the platysma muscle with very light four finger pressure. (Fig. 7.17) Three rows may be done from the top of the neck to the base of the neck so long as no pressure is applied in the area of the lymph nodes on the neck just above the clavicle.

25. Apply direct four finger pressure in toward the center of the neck on the sides just behind the ears (sternocleidomastoid) down to the base of the neck. (Fig. 7.18)

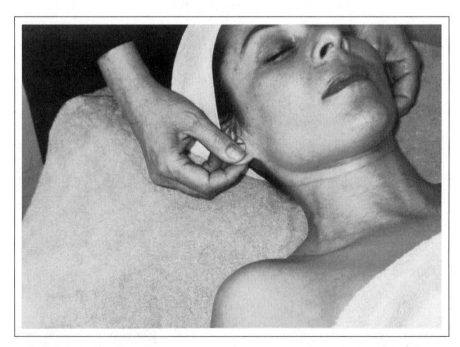

Fig. 7.16 Using thumb and first finger, apply equal pressure to the earlobes.

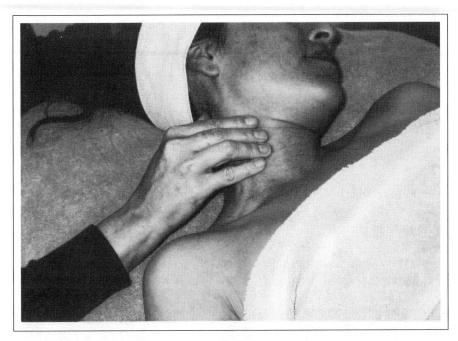

Fig. 7.17 Using four fingers, apply light pressure just next to the esophagus on the platysma muscle.

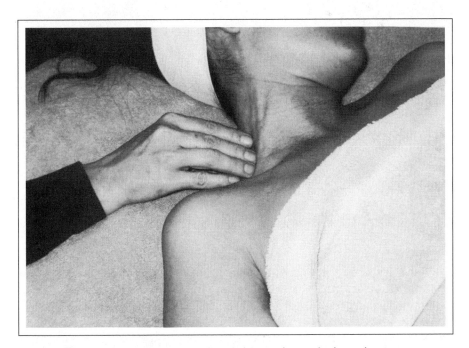

Fig. 7.18 Move toward the side of the neck just below the ears.

26. Apply thumb pressure to three *Tsubo* on top of shoulders and then on the center point at the top of the arm (top of deltoid muscle).

27. There will be approximately three rows for the chest from the top of the clavicle on both sides of the sternum between the ribs to the beginning of the breasts. No pressure is applied to the breasts themselves. Beginning just to the sides of the sternum apply full four finger pressure to approximately three rows out to the arm joint. Be sure the last row as you move down follows a line to the axilla. The last points are particularly relaxing and stress relieving. Do not apply pressure to lymph nodes in axilla area.

28. Final pressure on the chest will be done sideways with full hands on both sides of the sternum in a similar manner as done with the hands on the face.

The full facial treatment ends with a closing effleurage massage. The facial may then proceed as predetermined.

> **TARGET POINT**
>
> *Shiatsu* for the face accomplishes many things from relieving stress to increasing subsequent product absorption. It can be done as part of a regular facial or as a special service by itself.

Eye Treatment

Purpose

1. Relieves eye fatigue

2. Helps eyes lubricate and self-clarify (reduces redness)

3. Relaxes eyes to improve circulation and metabolism

4. Increases subsequent absorption of eye treatment products

5. May assist in relieving stress-related headaches

Technique

Keep in mind that the eyes are delicate and pressure must be very light. Proper pressure points in the eye area are located inside the ocular bone. When applying pressure to the upper eyelid, the pressure comes inside the bone just above the eyeball itself. When applying pressure to the lower lids, the fingers will actually be resting on the lashes and pressing on top of the lower ocular bone. Be sure to rest the back of the palms on the brow bone for added support. Both eyes will be done simultaneously so be careful to ensure even pressure on both sides.

1. Apply pressure with the middle or ring finger to the upper inner corner of eye just inside and under ocular bone.

2. Move to middle of upper eyelid; repeat pressure with same finger.

3. Move to outer corner of eye at junction of upper and lower eyelid; repeat pressure with same finger.

4. Apply pressure to temples with fingers or thumbs.

5. Repeat upper inner corner eyelid point.

6. Move to lower inner corner of eye at tear duct; apply lighter pressure with finger.

7. Move to lower middle lid; apply lighter pressure with same finger.

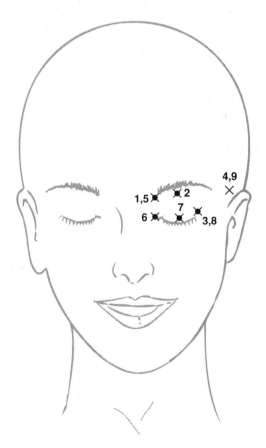

Eye treatment. Location of pressure points, step by step.

8. Move to outer corner of eye and apply similar pressure. (This point is the same location as for the outer corner of upper eyelid.)

9. Repeat temples.

TARGET POINT

The eye treatment alone is a very popular service because of its antistress and fatigue-relieving effects. This can easily be done in conjunction with a full eye treatment.

SUMMARY

Shiatsu for the face and head is a tremendously effective massage modality for relieving stress and tension. It provides great relaxation whether used as a partial treatment just around the eyes, for example, or over the entire face and head. The fact that it can be done in any order and for any part of the face makes it a most useful technique for the beginner and experienced technician.

REVIEW QUESTIONS

1. Is massage oil used for facial *Shiatsu* treatments in America?

2. Why would a *Shiatsu* treatment on the head be good to do?

3. How many groups are there in a full facial *Shiatsu* treatment (face, neck, chest)?

4. Normally in a facial treatment, what areas are done with the thumbs?

5. What does *Shiatsu* in an eye treatment do?

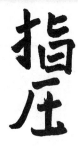

CHAPTER 8

Shiatsu for the Full Body: Hand/Arm, Foot/Leg, and Back Treatments

In addition to the five opening statements for chapter 7, there are some additional considerations to be kept in mind when doing *Shiatsu* on the body.

1. The already licensed massage therapist will have a good working knowledge of the musculature and anatomy of the body. The esthetician normally doesn't have that knowledge so cannot perform *Shiatsu* on the body without some additional training. It's important to at least know main muscle groups and how to do effleurage, so a practical course in massage may be necessary.

2. Although *Shiatsu* for the body is similar in that the specific order may vary according to the need, if the full body is being done, the normal recommended order will be as follows: Front side of the body—foot, leg, other foot and leg, hand, arm, other hand and arm, head, chest, shoulders. Then back side of the body—sole of foot, leg, other foot and leg, head, shoulders, upper arms, back.

3. In a full body treatment, about thirty-five minutes will be needed for the front side and twenty-five minutes for the back side.

4. Since there are many different sizes of bodies and technician hands, it's impossible to describe exactly how many points or rows are done on the body. For simplicity, generally do three points each on smaller areas, eight points each on larger areas, and sixteen points along the spine.

5. For most areas the thumbs will be used in an overlapping manner, but the four finger vice-grip technique may also be used on some smaller areas such as the back of the upper arm.

6. As you move from one area of the body to another be aware of the client's comfort level. The amount of pressure should be very light in certain areas such as the back of the knees and inner thighs. Pressure on the back may be much greater.

7. Always begin and end each area with effleurage.

8. Although already discussed, do not do *Shiatsu* on any areas of phlebitis or varicose veins, and be very cautious on a diabetic due to the predisposition to bruising.

TARGET POINT

Shiatsu for the body is more effective with a good knowledge of the muscular structure. If you are not a massage therapist, it would be wise to take a practical massage course before attempting to do *Shiatsu.*

BODY SHIATSU

Front Side

Purpose

1. *Shiatsu* relieves stress and tension in legs and arms.

2. Knees and ankles that are prone to water retention are relieved and the circulation is improved.

3. Circulation to the hands and feet is improved making the skin tone better, increasing nail growth, and providing an overall feeling of relaxation.

4. Stress and tension are relieved as the head, chest, and shoulders are done.

TARGET POINT

Body *Shiatsu* probably goes the furthest in relieving stress. The back in particular is a core relaxation area for the body.

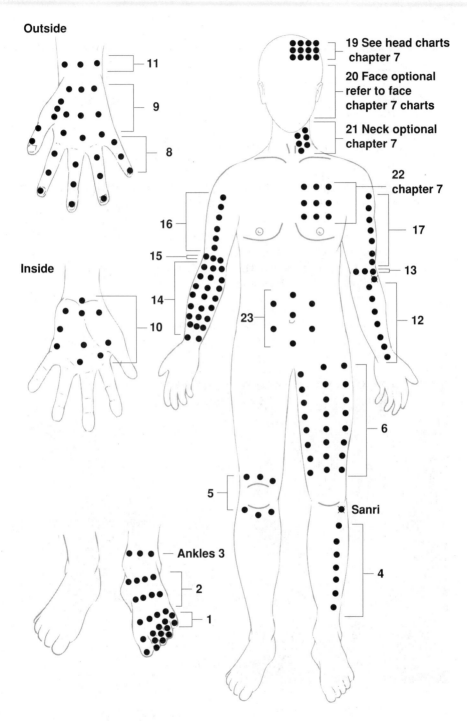

Body Shiatsu for the front side, noting pressure points.

Technique

Legs

1. Normally beginning with the foot of the left leg, starting with the little toe, pressure is applied with the thumb and first finger on the top and the sides between each joint of the toes. Keep pressure equal on both the thumb and finger. Work from the top/bottom of the tip of the toe inward to the base of the toe. (Fig. 8.2) The little toe and big toe normally have only two joints where the other toes have three. Do not apply pressure on the joints.

2. Moving from the toes to the top of the foot, pressure will be applied in four rows between the metatarsals and tarsals (bones of the foot to the ankle). Apply pressure to approximately three points between the base of the toe and the ankle in each row beginning at the outer side of the foot. Pressure is applied only to the top of the foot. (Fig. 8.3) The soles of the foot will be done later when the client is lying on the stomach.

3. Ankles: This can be a step by itself or included with step two. Apply pressure in the center and inside and outside of the ankle at the midpoint between the foot and calf where the ankle bends.

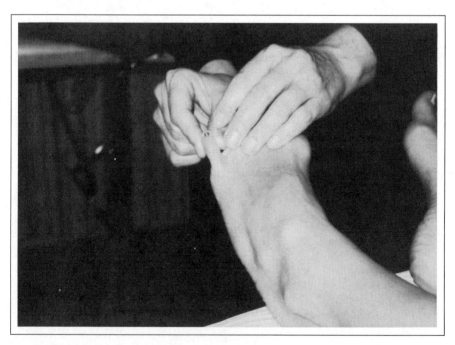

Fig. 8.2 Apply pressure to the sides of the little toe. Remember, do not apply pressure to the joints.

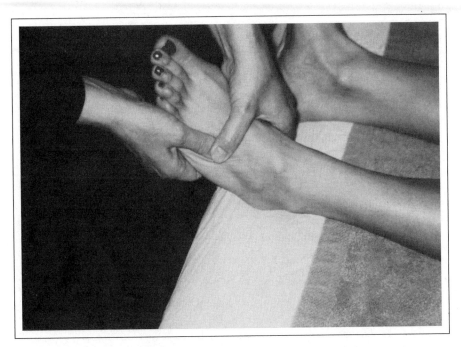

Fig. 8.3 Apply pressure to the top of the foot.

4. Using thumbs overlapped, apply pressure up the calf of the leg just outside the tibia (bone on front of calf). (Fig. 8.4) As you near the knee the angle of the line will veer to the outside where the final point is reached about three fingers below the knee and almost one inch to the outside. This last point is called the *Sanri* and is thought to be a central *Tsubo* for the general well-being of the entire body.

5. Apply pressure to three points below and above the knee.

6. The thigh is done in three rows; the top, then inside, then outside. The leg is kept straight to do the eight points up the center of the thigh (center of quadriceps). Then bend the leg out in order to use careful pressure up the inside of the thigh right in the middle. There is a very obvious dent between the muscles, and your hands should follow right along the dent to the base of the leg. The leg is then straightened out and pressure is applied from the knee up the outer side of the leg also between the muscles to the base of the leg. Sometimes it's more convenient for the technician to turn facing the leg from the side and apply thumb overlapping thumb pressure up the thigh.

7. Repeat steps one to six on the right leg.

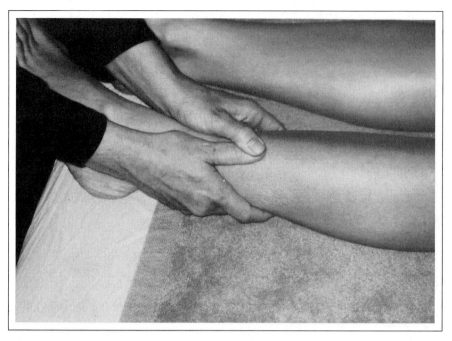

Fig. 8.4 Overlap thumbs and apply pressure up the calf of the leg.

Arms

1. Moving to the fingers of the left hand, perform pressure between the joints of the top/bottom and sides of the fingers in a similar manner as with the toes. Start with the little finger working in to the thumbs. Do not forget to do the thumbs. Use thumb and first fingers to do the fingers of the client. (Fig. 8.5)

2. The back and front of the hands will be done at this point. First apply pressure on the metacarpels and carpels from the little finger to the first finger in the same manner as for the feet. Four rows will be done with three points per row. The last row is the row from the base of the thumb to the wrist, so there are actually only three rows corresponding to the fingers themselves. (Fig. 8.6)

3. Turn to the inside of the hand and spread the fingers by inserting your little fingers between the thumb/first finger and the little finger/ring finger and open the hand of the client. Apply pressure from the center of the base of the middle finger directly down the center of the hand (three points) and then follow around the padded part of the palm doing about six to eight points ending at the fleshy part of the palm at the base of the thumb. (Fig. 8.7) Effleurage hands again and turn to the back of the hand.

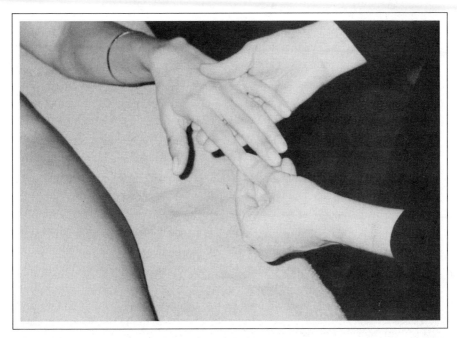

Fig. 8.5 Using the thumb and first finger, apply pressure to the top of the fingers (as done with the toes).

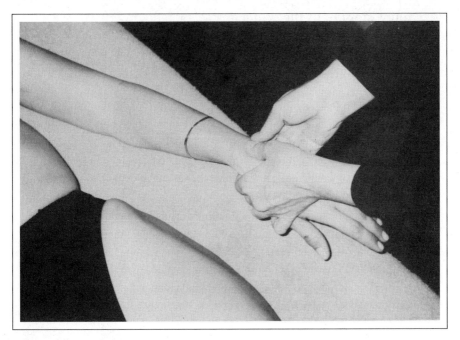

Fig. 8.6 Apply pressure from the base of the thumb to the wrist.

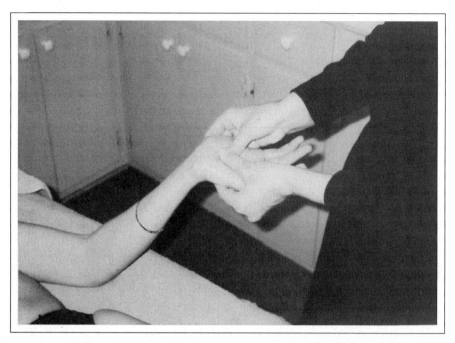

Fig. 8.7 Apply pressure to the palm just below the middle finger.

4. Apply pressure to the center, inside, outside of wrist. (Fig. 8.8)

5. Work up the lower arm between the extensor muscles from the wrist to slightly below the elbow and slightly outside. There is a similar *Sanri* point on the lower arm to the same point on the calves of the legs. (Fig. 8.9)

6. Apply pressure on the middle, inside, outside of elbow. Turn to inside of lower arm.

7. Apply pressure in three rows up the inside lower arm, middle, inside, outside. Support the arm with your arm or place the arm on the bed to apply pressure.

8. Apply lighter pressure to the middle, inside, outside of inner elbow. (Fig. 8.10)

9. Apply pressure in one row up the center of the upper arm. Turn to back of arm. (Fig. 8.11)

10. Apply pressure to outer arm while supporting client's arm or putting it on the bed.

11. Repeat steps one to ten on the right hand and arm.

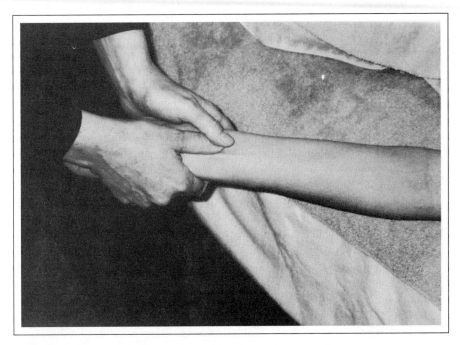

Fig. 8.8 Move around the wrist, continuing to apply pressure.

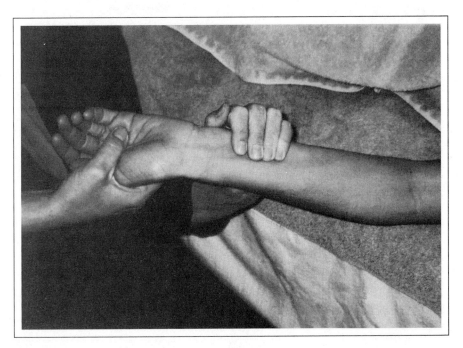

Fig. 8.9 Begin to work up the arm, applying constant pressure.

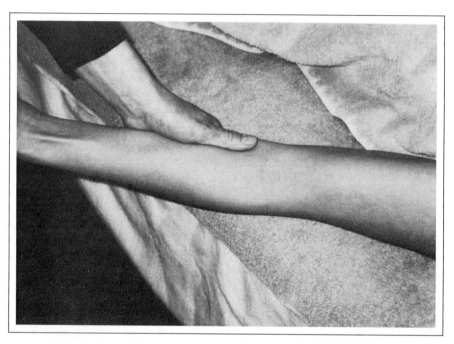

Fig. 8.10 Apply pressure to the outside of the elbow.

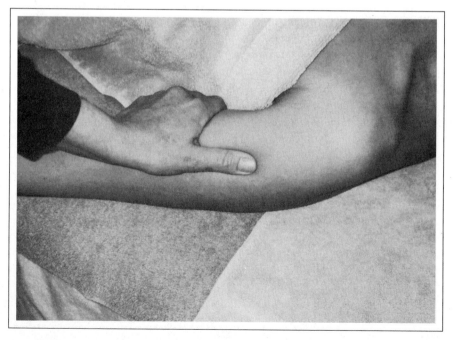

Fig. 8.11 Work up the center of the arm, applying pressure.

Head, Neck, Chest

1. Move to the top of the head and apply pressure to the main head *Tsubo* on the crown with the pressure aiming toward the tip of the feet. (Fig. 8.12) Then other head points may be done either by the full side hand vice-grip positioning or one at a time by the thumb overlap thumb technique. (See chapter 7 for points.) This will depend on how much time you have. Do only the top of the head. The back of the head will be done when the client reverses position.

2. The face may be done as an option at this point. (Follow steps from chapter 7.) Normally the face is not done in a body *Shiatsu* treatment. Facial *Shiatsu* is generally sold as a type of facial treatment. But you may choose to just do a few strategic points such as the forehead, temples, and inner corner of eyes.

3. The neck may be done just as shown in chapter 7 if desired or you may skip from top of head to the chest.

4. The three rows of the chest are then done as shown in chapter 7.

5. If desired, very light pressure may be done on the stomach/abdominal area. Most often it is better to use the palms of the hands and

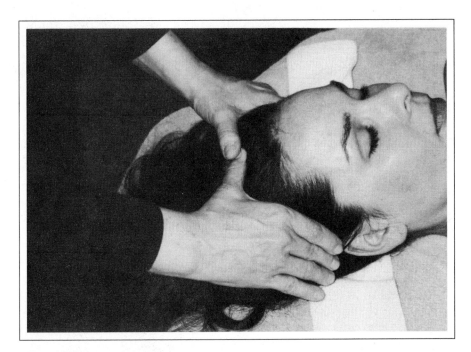

Fig. 8.12 Apply pressure to the main head *Tsubo*.

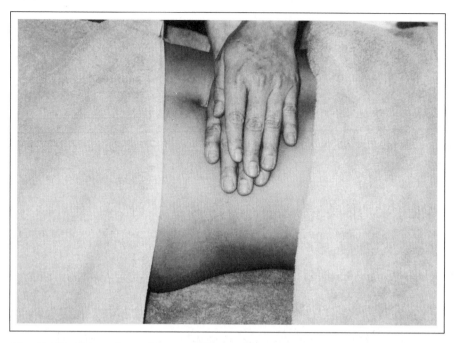

Fig. 8.13 Using the palms, apply pressure around the navel.

apply pressure to four to six points in a clockwise direction around the navel, starting directly above the navel just below the rib cage (solar plexus area). (Fig. 8.13) Stomach *Shiatsu* is rarely done in most American beauty-related body treatments.

To close, after the final effleurage is done, remove any excess massage oil, apply finishing body powder to the entire body, and polish. Then it is very nice to go over the arms and legs with the full thumb finger vice-grip over the towel/sheets. This is just a quick overall pressure to relax the client and prepare for rolling over onto the stomach.

Back Side of Body

Purpose

1. The back side is normally the most relaxing part of any massage treatment, and *Shiatsu* is no different. Although pressure to the back of the legs has to be lighter, greater pressure is exerted to the back for greater relaxation of the client.

2. *Shiatsu* on the back tremendously relieves stress and fatigue.

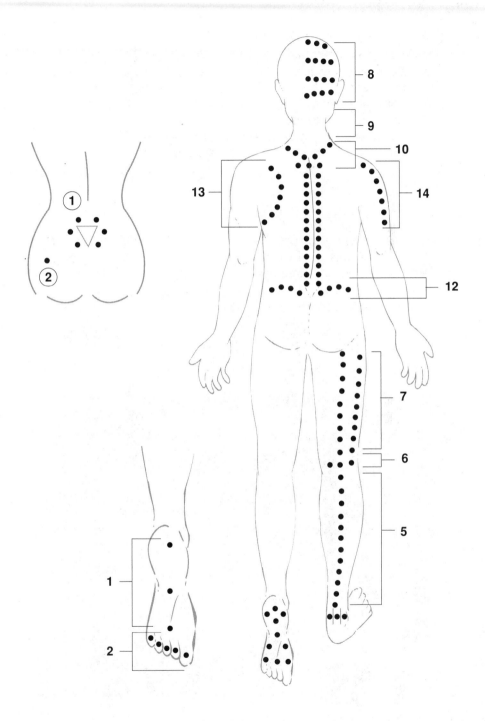

Back side, noting pressure points.

3. The knots and lumps in the shoulders from lactic acid buildup are relieved by *Shiatsu* of the back.

4. Without doing the bottoms of the feet for relief of any medical condition, keep in mind that all meridians start at the top of the head and end in the feet. Think of the meridians as paths going from the head to the feet. A good *Shiatsu* of the feet will work wonders for the circulation and well-being of the entire body. *Shiatsu* of the feet can also be equated to reflexology but without specific concentration on points for curative purposes.

Technique

Legs

1. Starting at the bottom of the feet, you may do a very brief *Shiatsu* by applying pressure from the top of the foot in the center to the base of the foot in three points. However, for a full, deep-relaxing treatment, it is good to do more. If so, begin by applying pressure to the large pad of each toe. (Fig. 8.15)

2. Do pressure down the center row of the foot with deep relaxing pressure (approximately three points). (Fig. 8.16)

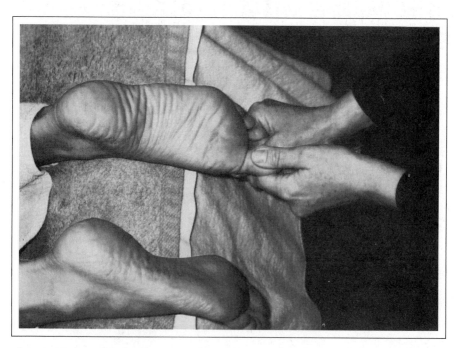

Fig. 8.15 Apply pressure to the large pad of each toe.

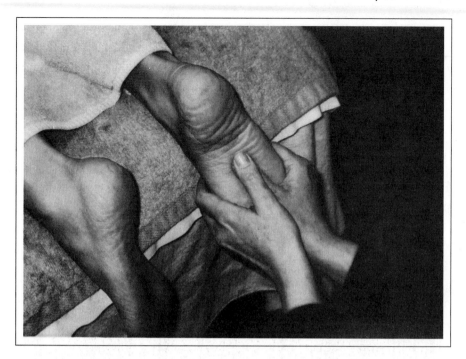

Fig. 8.16 Apply pressure down the center row of the foot.

3. Similarly to the hands, apply pressure on about eight points working from the last midpoint on the heel around the foot to the same midpoint again.

4. Apply pressure to the center of the ankle, then inside, outside.

5. Apply pressure from the ankle to the popliteal space (behind the knee) concentrating the heavier pressure in the main body of the calf (gastrocnemius muscle). There should be about eight points working up the center of the lower leg.

6. Apply much lighter pressure to the center, inside, outside of the popliteal space. Be very careful in this area and avoid entirely if varicose veins exist or if too tender to client.

7. The upper leg will be done in two rows, one row of about eight points up the center of the thigh and the second row on the outer thigh. Moving to the side and applying pressure in a thumb overlap thumb manner is effective for the outer thigh. (Fig. 8.17)

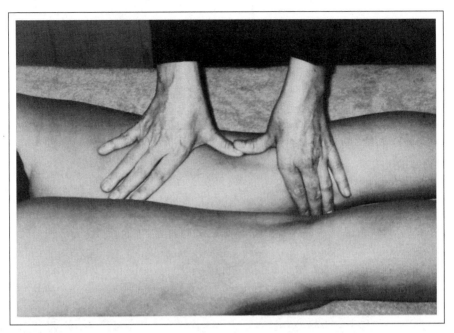

Fig. 8.17 Apply lighter pressure working up back of thigh.

Head/Neck

1. Apply pressure to the main crown point and then three points down the back of the head to the occipital. (Fig. 8.18) If time allows, you may do three points in five rows as discussed in chapter 7. The main row and then base of the occipital are the more strategic points. Again, the base of the occipital should be done with the fingers in a deep lifting manner.

2. Apply pressure to the sides of the back of the neck with the thumb four finger grip technique. (Fig. 8.19)

Shoulders/Back

1. The top of the shoulders should be effleuraged again before and in between concentrated points on the upper shoulder (trapezius) area. A good five minutes should be spent on the shoulders if necessary. Although only a few points are shown in the diagram, the entire upper trapezius is prone to stress and fatigue and you will find many tender areas that should be worked. But do not apply pressure to the point of discomfort.

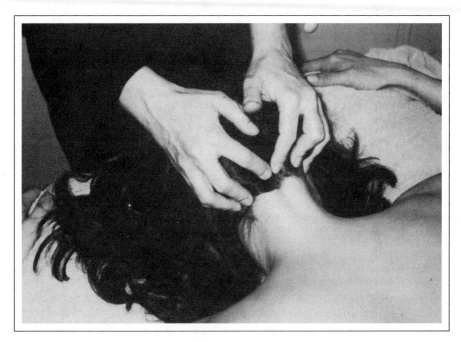

Fig. 8.18 Apply pressure to the main crown point and then down the back of the head to the occipital.

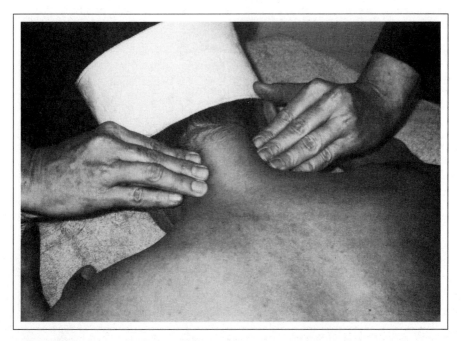

Fig. 8.19 Apply pressure to the sides of the neck.

2. Apply pressure to approximately sixteen points down the spine to the upper buttocks area. Pressure may be applied by both thumbs side by side on both sides of the spine at the same time if desired. (Fig. 8.20) However, due to the potential for stress on the thumbs, you may choose to overlap the thumbs and work sideways down one side of the spine and go around to the other side of the client to repeat the process down the other side.

3. Apply pressure with the base of the palms to the base of the back and upper buttock area. (Fig. 8.21) There will be one row of about three pressure points.

4. Moving back up to the scapula (shoulder blades) with a full back effleurage technique will position you well for the final *Shiatsu* area on the back. The *Tsubo* around the shoulder blades often carry a lot of stress so apply pressure to about eight points following the anatomy of the shoulder blade from the top around to the base at the side of the client. (Fig. 8.22) Move to the other side and repeat on the other shoulder blade. If the *Tsubo* are difficult to locate, you may ask the client to put an arm behind the back to help you define the line by stroking the area. Then move the client's arm back to a comfortable position and apply pressure.

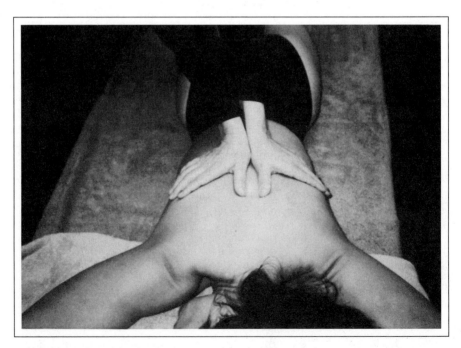

Fig 8.20 Work down the spine.

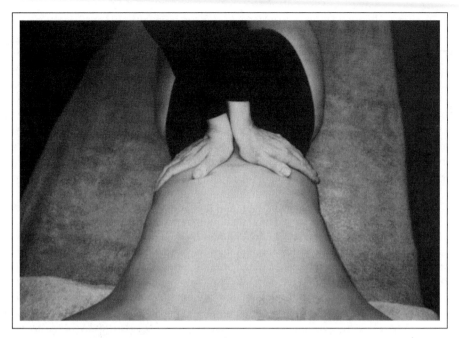

Fig. 8.21 With the base of the palms, apply pressure to the base of the back and the upper buttocks area.

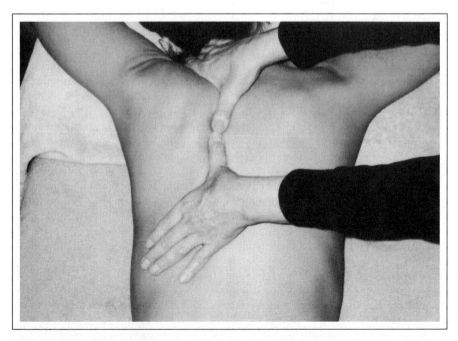

Fig. 8.22 Apply pressure to the shoulder blade.

5. Even though the upper arms were done on the front side, it provides a very relaxing and comfortable ending to the *Shiatsu* to repeat the upper arm/top of outer shoulder points (approximately eight points) once more working from the top of the shoulder out to about the middle of the upper arm.

(Note: Generally in America the buttocks are not done. However, if desired, apply pressure across the top of the buttocks at the base of the back as done in step three. Then apply pressure around the coccyx bone in a clockwise manner. The final point will be a deep pressure from the side at the dimple in the buttocks with the thumb overlap thumb technique.)

To close the treatment, the final effleurage is done on the back, shoulders, and upper arms. The residue of any massage oil is removed and finishing body powder applied and buffed. The client is then covered and a quick open full hand pressure is applied to the head, neck, shoulders, back, and on down the legs to the feet where final pressure is applied with the base of the palms of the hands.

At this point the treatment is completed and the client should be awake. The lights should be turned up and the client rolled over onto the back and then helped to a sitting position. A robe is given to the client and a short discussion of home care product needs might take place. Every client needs body lotions, special soaps, exfoliants, bath oils, etc., and this is the ideal time to sell the client what's needed. This should be done at this time to accomplish two things at once.

1. The client could be a little light-headed and you don't want to rush. This allows the client to stabilize. Giving the client juice or water at this time is also good.

2. While doing the treatment you should have been able to determine at least two to three products the client should be using on the body at home. This is the ideal time to explain the products. Then while the client is dressing, you are able to prepare the products and total the bill.

TARGET POINT

Finish a full body *Shiatsu* treatment with the application of a good body polish by using finishing powder. This enhances the treatment and gives a healthy glow to the skin.

Back Treatment

Purpose

1. Back facials are a very popular and well-known treatment in the salon. In the same manner, a back *Shiatsu* treatment can be a quick but very stress-relieving opportunity for your clients.

2. Everyone has stress and lactic acid buildup. A treatment just for the back can draw the client to other body treatments in the salon.

3. A back treatment takes very little time and can even be done in ten minutes over clothes anywhere in the salon.

Technique

1. Open with overall effleurage of the shoulders and back. Then apply pressure to the upper shoulders area in two or three rows of three points keeping close to the spinal column.

2. Apply pressure to approximately sixteen points down the spinal column as explained in the section for back on the full body.

3. Apply pressure with the base of the palms to the base of the back/upper buttocks. There will be one row of about three points.

4. Apply pressure around the scapula on each side of the spine (locating points described in back section of full body).

5. Apply thumb four finger grip down the upper arms.

6. Finish with final full back effleurage, remove any oil residue, and buff with body finishing powder. Cover back with towel and apply palm pressure down the sides of the spine, out the base of the back, and squeeze the upper arms.

TARGET POINT

There is no part of the body that shows such relief from stress as the back area and just a back treatment alone will go far in developing more business for *Shiatsu* and other body treatments.

Hand/Arm Treatment

Purpose

1. *Shiatsu* can dramatically enhance a regular manicure and set you apart with a special draw to build business.

2. Clients carry more stress in hands and arms than is normally thought. *Shiatsu* in this area is very relaxing and stress relieving.

3. *Shiatsu* will allow you to convert your manicure into a more so-phisticated treatment along with other day-spa-type treatments and you can charge extra for it.

Technique

1. The technique will basically be the same as in a full body treatment, the main difference being that you will be sitting up and holding the client's hand/arm while working. *Shiatsu* for the hands will be done exactly as described in the full body treatment. Apply pressure on the fingers, back of hand, inside of hand.

2. Apply pressure to the outside then inside of the lower arm as shown in the full body treatment while supporting the arm with the other hand. Pressure will be done with one hand while the other hand supports the lower arm.

3. Apply pressure to the inside and outside three points of the elbow.

4. The upper arm is a little more difficult. You will hold the arm by the elbow with the forearm balanced over your arm. The other hand will apply pressure to the inner and outer sides of the upper arm. It may·work well to use the thumb four finger grip if the arm is small enough.

5. Effleurage and continue with predetermined treatment.

Foot/Leg Treatment

Purpose

1. A more sophisticated foot and leg treatment will enhance your normal pedicure and set you above your competition.

2. As has already been stated, the feet are the end points of the merid-ian system and a *Shiatsu* treatment for the feet alone will make a client feel great, relieve stress, and help the client relax.

3. Adding *Shiatsu* to a pedicure can convert a regular pedicure into a sophisticated day-spa treatment that is chargeable.

Technique

1. The difference in the foot/leg treatment from the full body lies in the fact that you will be treating the client from a sitting

position, and you will be seated in front of the client. The toes and top of the foot are done the same. After this is completed, lift the foot a little more and apply pressure to the points listed in the full body treatment on the sole of the foot only. Do not repeat the toes.

2. Apply pressure to the top, inside, outside of the ankles.

3. Apply pressure with a thumb over thumb technique up the calf. It is wise to hold the calf with both hands and gradually slide up to apply pressure. The back of the calf will be done with the fingers in the thumb four finger grip technique working from the bottom of the leg up to the knee.

4. Apply pressure to the three points below the knee.

5. Effleurage again and continue with the predetermined treatment.

TARGET POINT

There is nothing better than adding a little *Shiatsu* to a manicure or pedicure to impress your client. If you decide to do a full-fledged treatment with *Shiatsu* it becomes a new chargeable service as well.

SUMMARY

With so much emphasis on well-being these days, *Shiatsu* is the ideal stress-relieving treatment. It may be used in back treatments to reduce the accumulation of tension and lactic acid very effectively. *Shiatsu* alone, or combined with manicures and pedicures, makes that treatment much more pleasing and unique. And the ultimate, of course, is the use of *Shiatsu* as a full body treatment in conjunction with other treatments, massage, or entirely alone. The versatility of *Shiatsu* in body treatments will add to any other salon service from a client satisfaction standpoint and from a profit standpoint for the salon owner.

REVIEW QUESTIONS

1. How long does it take to do *Shiatsu* on the front side of a client and then on the back side if doing a full body treatment?

2. Name a few of the reasons to do *Shiatsu* on the body.

3. Is it safe to do *Shiatsu* over varicose veins or on a diabetic? Why?

4. What is the marketing value of a *Shiatsu* back treatment?

5. What good does it do to add *Shiatsu* to a manicure or pedicure?

PART III

THE BUSINESS OF SHIATSU

CHAPTER 9

Marketing Shiatsu Services

The structure and operational aspects of *Shiatsu* should now be quite clear. From a technical aspect, there's no better way to master this wonderful and effective ancient art but with practice, practice, practice. Beyond practice, it must also be clear to you that the best technique in the world cannot build the business by itself. It's certainly an important part but cannot be the only sustaining factor. Although it's good to know that if you give a great treatment to a client that person may go out and tell many relatives and friends who will subsequently come into the business for a treatment themselves, waiting for this to build your business could be very disappointing as well as defeating.

You must take a proactive approach to build this exciting new service. It's very easy to think that because you've spent a lot of time learning the service that you're automatically telling enough people about it, but it really doesn't work that way. Word of mouth is, of course, a good marketing technique, but it's only one facet. Let's discuss the marketing approach to *Shiatsu* in more detail.

TARGET POINT

Practicing *Shiatsu* is important to become an expert, but marketing the service will make it known in your business.

DEVELOPING A MENU

Shiatsu may be offered in a number of ways but the two most common ways follow.

Small Complimentary Bits of Shiatsu

You can incorporate small bits or area parts of *Shiatsu* into a regular service. For example, you may do a couple of special *Tsubo* around the eyes and temple in a regular facial. If this is added into a facial, then you would not normally charge extra for it. But when doing it as a complimentary part of a regular treatment, it's always wise to talk about it and offer the client the opportunity for a full *Shiatsu* treatment. Remember, bits of complimentary *Shiatsu* can be added to facial treatments, body massage, manicure/pedicure, or even a shampoo. Aside from the fact that you're doing these bits to relax and make your client appreciate the regular treatment more, you should be using this opportunity to sell the client a full treatment.

Full Chargeable Shiatsu Treatment

Naturally, the real goal is to be able to offer a full service of *Shiatsu* on a charge basis. For example, if you're giving a facial and want to make it a *Shiatsu* facial, you'll spend about thirty minutes on the massage and *Shiatsu* part of that facial making the whole hour facial about one and a half hours long. The charge for this must be commensurate with the time and effort spent. Listed are some suggested treatments to offer and times normally needed to accomplish the service. Pricing will be discussed in the next section.

Shiatsu Scalp Treatment	15 minutes
Full Face *Shiatsu* Massage	30 minutes
Shiatsu Eye Treatment	15 minutes
Full *Shiatsu* Body Treatment	1 hour
Shiatsu Hand/Arm	15–30 minutes
Shiatsu Foot/Leg	15–30 minutes
Shiatsu Back Treatment	30 minutes

Always remember that even on a charge basis, *Shiatsu* can be an add-on to the regular treatment or charged for as a *Shiatsu* massage by itself. If doing the *Shiatsu* purely by itself, you'll need to charge full price but may discount it somewhat if adding it into another service already being done because it normally takes a little less time since the client is already set up and creams or oils are being used anyway.

TARGET POINT

Shiatsu may be done complimentary in small areas as part of the treatment, but it must also be offered as a separate and special service that is charged for.

PRICING THE SHIATSU SERVICE

Pricing is always a difficult issue because prices you can charge in New York or Aspen, Colorado, are most likely more than you can charge in Boise, Idaho, or Laramie, Wyoming. There are three factors that should be considered when adding a service and determining the price.

1. Determine a new service price based on your average per minute pricing for other services and prorate accordingly. For example, if your regular facial treatment sells for $60 and takes one hour, your per minute value is $1. Therefore, if you did a *Shiatsu* eye treatment and it took fifteen minutes, you could charge $15.

2. The new service should also have some excitement value or what I often call "exotic value." Certainly *Shiatsu* is somewhat exotic. You spent a great deal of time, money, and effort to learn it, so it also has some add-on value. So in addition to your per minute value, you may add a bit of an exotic charge. Perhaps with interesting music and presentation, you decide to offer that eye treatment for $20 instead of $15.

3. What the market will bear is another calculation you must consider. If you're the only person in town offering *Shiatsu*, you have a little more freedom to be pricey or to escalate your exotic value, but you don't want to price yourself out of the market. So in all issues of pricing, be sure to have a good feel for what your competition is doing, the value of your salon's name and reputation, etc. In some cases this will allow you to charge even more, but in some cases it may mean that you charge less.

So, in all pricing decisions, take all three of these points into consideration before finalizing your pricing. Remember, you must price this service. Just doing it for free forever is not fair to you or to the value of *Shiatsu* itself.

Once you have determined what *Shiatsu* services you'll offer and at what price, you need to market it!

TARGET POINT

Charge what is reasonable and allowable in your area by valuing your time per minute, adding a bit for the uniqueness, and keeping your prices within reason of your competition.

LITERATURE DEVELOPMENT

As stated already, it doesn't do you any good to have a great new service if you don't market it. Whenever you offer a new service, it needs to be given proper attention in your literature. You may not immediately print new salon price lists if you still have three thousand old ones to get rid of, but you need to make a special flyer to announce the service or offer an introductory special of some kind. In the case of *Shiatsu*, make it a great flyer. Spend the money for good paper and an interesting presentation. Use slightly oriental fonts. Give that flyer a real flair, something that attracts the client's interest. Then when your salon is ready for new brochures, be sure *Shiatsu* is on the new menu of services. But while you're waiting, you're building business for the service from day one.

You may want to write a newsletter to your clients including technical information to help them understand why they should come in for the service. Education and information on the direct benefits to the clients will go far to encourage interest. Even if you don't currently mail your clients a newsletter, send a letter out to each client introducing *Shiatsu* and its benefits. The mailing will certainly generate interest and talk and, if accompanied with some kind of promotion, will develop new business.

TARGET POINT

You can have the greatest service but if nobody knows, what good is it? Make a good brochure, flyer, or newsletter to get the word out there.

PRESS COVERAGE

It doesn't matter what city or town you're located in, the addition of *Shiatsu* services is a newsworthy event. After your class, immediately go home and develop a press release to send to your local newspapers and local area publications. You may even send the release to the radio and TV stations. There is no guarantee that the editors and newspeople will ever use the release but they may. You never know when the editor has a hole in the paper and needs a filler. Or perhaps, the disc jockey on the radio had experienced *Shiatsu* somewhere and shows interest in your service.

If you write a cover letter with the release, you might want to invite the editor or publisher in for a complimentary treatment. If by chance you are written up, the potential business from even the briefest mention might shock you. If you have a photo of you doing the service or with

SHIATSU PRESS RELEASE (Sample)

When writing your release, remember the following:

1. Always write in third person.

2. Send 5×7 or 8×12 black-and-white glossy photograph.

3. Never mention your name or your salon name more than twice.

4. Never mention prices.

5. Invite the beauty/fashion editor to your salon for a free treatment.

FOR IMMEDIATE RELEASE: New Oriental Massage

Contact: Name
          Address
          Phone

"MY SALON" NOW OFFERS
SHIATSU ORIENTAL MASSAGE

Double Space

Jane Doe of My Salon has just returned from a ____ day intensive workshop on Shiatsu Oriental Massage. Shiatsu is an extremely effective massage technique based on Chinese medical concepts. The instructor, Erica Miller, graduated from the Imai Shiatsu Massage School in Tokyo, Japan. This advanced treatment can benefit stress, pain (headaches), and relaxation.

Shiatsu is now being offered at:

          Your Salon
          Your Address
          Your Town

your instructor, something visual that will add to the newsworthiness, your chances of being published are greater.

If you are involved in a large salon business and already employ a public relations (PR) agent for media coverage, then let that person know so he/she can get the releases and PR coverage out. The reality of press coverage is that you never know when it will be printed, but when it is you will benefit far greater than the amount of time and energy spent in the preparation and mailing of the release.

Always be prepared to offer the editors and prominent people offering you the press coverage a complimentary treatment. There is an additional advantage if that person comes into your salon. You will get to know the press on a more personal basis, they will remember your salon, and they may then remember to consider you a resource for future quotes on beauty-related articles. The long-term benefits for your business may go far beyond the scope of the *Shiatsu* release itself. Always remember that any editorial exposure you get is not only free but also generally considered more effective than a paid ad.

TARGET POINT

Free editorial coverage with press releases sometimes provides a better response than a paid ad. It's worth the effort to do press releases.

ADVERTISING AND PROMOTIONS

There is always value in running an ad for the launch of a new, interesting and unique service such as *Shiatsu*. But in the ad, be sure you target the copy to the benefit of the client, not just to the technical aspect of what *Shiatsu* does. The public doesn't really care much beyond the personal benefit. It's wise in your ad and service launch to have some kind of promotion to kick it off. There are mainly two kinds of promotions.

Service Discount

When launching a new service it is sometimes good to offer an introductory discount for a specified period of time. Another method is to include the new service with a regular treatment at a reduced introductory price. This will encourage the client to go ahead and try the service while in the salon. When discounting a new service, 10-15 percent is normally adequate, but, again, you need to take your competition into consideration.

Gift with Purchase

In this author's opinion, a gift with purchase is by far the more preferable option. The advantage is that you not only have the client in the salon receiving the service you wanted but you also get a product in the client's hand to try at home. It may seem that you're giving away actual cost of a product versus your time, but the reality is that you will value the product to the client at the normal retail price but your wholesale cost on it is normally half that amount.

Additionally, when you give a service away, you're also giving away time that might have been spent on another paying client who might have purchased a product too. And the most valuable reason to give a home care product is to solidify the salon treatment with more effectiveness. If the product does what you want it to, then you build client loyalty as well.

But when giving a product away, be sure the blend makes sense. Why give a lipstick as a gift for a body massage? This doesn't make sense, and what do you do when a man opts for the massage? In the case of a *Shiatsu* treatment, depending on the area you're working on, give a product for that area's real need. For example, if you did a full body *Shiatsu* treatment and realized that the client had very dry skin, how about a conditioning body lotion? Or, if you had used oil and finished the treatment with a great finishing powder, how about giving a finishing powder?

There are many different promotional items that can be given but be sure you maximize the value to both you and the client. Remember, don't give away products you're trying to get rid of. That has no residual meaning or value to either you or the client. Give products that will build future business because that is the entire idea. If you have old products you want to get rid of, then do it in a different way such as making a contribution.

You can tie any number of home care retail products to the new *Shiatsu* service, develop a series package of three or six repeat treatments, and increase the value of the gift with purchase to balance the mix well.

Don't forget the benefit to be gleaned from having your clients promote the new *Shiatsu* treatments for you. Offer a special where if your existing client brings three new clients, she gets the service complimentary or receives a free product. You may create any number of great promotions along this idea.

If your salon or day spa offers various packages of different treatments, be sure to put the new *Shiatsu* service in a package with older, very high selling, popular services. This way, the person automatically experiences the new treatment even though the main goal of purchasing the package may have been for some other service. It will increase consumer awareness as well.

TARGET POINT

A combination of great technique, good menu development, proper literature, and press coverage will ensure the success of a launch of a new service such as *Shiatsu*. This success comes from thinking as a businessperson just as much as thinking as a technician!

SUMMARY

Bottom line to this whole chapter is that if you don't aggressively market your new *Shiatsu* services nobody else will, and they won't necessarily take off by themselves. *Shiatsu* is a wonderful and proven beneficial treatment in so many different areas of the salon. But if you don't push it, the benefits are lost. So go out there, practice, and build a great *Shiatsu* business.

REVIEW QUESTIONS

1. Is a good technique sufficient to build the *Shiatsu* business?

2. How much should you charge for a *Shiatsu* treatment?

3. Why is a brochure or menu important to promote *Shiatsu*?

4. Should you give *Shiatsu* treatments to anyone free?

5. What kind of a gift with purchase is good with *Shiatsu*?

Answers to
Review Questions

CHAPTER 1

1. Upon what is Ayurvedic medicine based?

   Ayurvedic medicine means "science of life." It is a system of medicine that combines natural therapies with a highly personalized approach to the treatment of disease.

2. Chinese medicine includes what three elements?

   Moxibustion, acupuncture, herbal medicine.

3. What is the meridian system?

   The energy pathway system of the body comprising twelve longitudinal channels is called the meridian system.

4. For what is Hippocrates known?

   He is often considered the Father of Modern Medicine, but is perhaps best known for the charter of medical conduct known as the Hippocratic oath.

5. When did Chinese medicine enter Japan?

   Chinese medicine entered Japan through Korea around 458 B.C.

6. What does the word *Shiatsu* mean?

   Finger pressure.

7. What do *yin* and *yang* represent?

   Yin and *yang* represent the concept of the entire universe being in harmony. *Yin* is the negative or female principle representing the earth and dark. *Yang* is the positive or male principle representing the heavens and light.

CHAPTER 2

1. From where did the term *reflex action* come?

   The term was coined by Dr. Marshall Hall (1790-1857) to connote the relationship between the brain, spinal cord, and other parts of the body. His research on the subject of reflex action on the nervous system led to the use of the term.

2. What did English researchers Sir Henry Head and Sir Charles Sherrington contribute to the concept of reflex action?

They were doing research on neurology and connected the skin with organs. They confirmed that there was a link between the brain, spinal cord, and reflex pathways that would control functions of the entire body. Their work came to be taught in medical schools.

3. Who developed the theory that pressure application incited various changes in the body?

Dr. Alfons Cornelius in his book *Druckpunkte, or Pressure Points, Their Origin and Significance* developed this theory.

4. Who is considered the Father of Zone Therapy?

The Father of Zone Therapy is Dr. William Fitzgerald.

5. Essentially, what is zone therapy?

Zone therapy is the concept whereby direct pressure on certain areas of the body would produce an analgesic effect in a corresponding part.

6. With what is Eunice Ingham credited?

She is credited with furthering the concept of zone therapy into a therapy whereby application of pressure would not only produce an analgesic effect but would also stimulate the body to heal itself. She concentrated her therapy on the feet.

7. For what important legislation is Tokujiro Namikoshi responsible?

He pressed for legislation in Japan that would recognize *Shiatsu* as a viable science and ultimately developed a licensing board.

8. Do *Shiatsu* experts and reflexologists practice medicine?

No they do not. Although the history is based on medical practices, these professionals practice in America for good health and well-being.

9. Is there any validity to the concept of Chinese meridians?

There is still difficulty proving the validity to many Western scientists, but much has been done to validate the therapy. As a couple of examples, Dr. Kim Bong and a team of researchers in Korea found evidence that there may be a system of ductlike tubes corresponding to the paths of the original Chinese meridians. Dr. Robert O. Becke and Maria Reichmanis, a biophysicist, under a grant from the National Institutes of Health (1970s) were able to prove that electrical currents did indeed flow along the ancient Chinese meridians and that some of the points were also scientifically measurable.

CHAPTER 3

1. What is *Ki?*

   Ki is considered the universal energy that flows within the body through a pattern or matrix that links the body's vital organs with all the other body parts as well as linking the body parts to all environmental forces of nature.

2. What was central to the understanding of the ancient Chinese philosophy, science, and culture?

   To the Chinese, all the myriad things in heaven obey the law of *Ki* balance. The harmony of *Ki* provides harmony to all aspects of the universe including the human body.

3. Discuss some attributes of *yin* and *yang* overall.

   The concept of *yin* and *yang* represent the harmony and equal balance of all things in the universe. *Yin* represents the negative, dark, female principles and *yang* represents the positive, light, male concepts. These concepts are interdependent and complementary. When one is up the other is down.

4. What are some aspects of *yin* and *yang* in the body?

   See page 23 for chart.

5. What are meridians? What is a *Tsubo* and where is it located?

   Meridians are the energy pathways in the body. *Tsubo* are motor points located along the meridians that connect one area of the body to an organ or other system along the corresponding meridian.

6. How many meridians are normally considered in *Shiatsu* treatment?

   Normally twelve channels are considered for *Shiatsu.*

7. What is the difference in the energy flow between *yin* and *yang?*

   Yin energy flows up from the feet to the chest and out the fingertips. *Yang* energy flows downward from the hands to the head and down to the feet.

8. What are the Five Elements?

   The Five Elements are wood, fire, earth, metal, water.

9. What are the three results of *Shiatsu* treatment?

Shiatsu treatment can self-regulate pain and discomfort through the natural release of endorphins; increase energy to the entire body, and relax the body while relieving fatigue and stress.

10. How can overall harmony be achieved?

Overall harmony can be achieved through the concept of the *yin-yang* balance, restoring the overall harmony of the entire person by invigorating the skin, stimulating the various circulatory systems, balancing the endocrine and digestive systems, and facilitating the normal functioning of the organs.

CHAPTER 4

1. What is an example of an interesting difference between the cultures of America and Japan?

One interesting difference is the hugging and kissing done in the West but massage being performed between members of the family in Japan when they don't hug and kiss and we don't massage.

2. How is massage (and *Shiatsu*) viewed in the American home versus the Japanese home?

Massage is a normal and natural thing in Japan. Most children massage their parents and other family members in Japan whereas massage is not commonly practiced in American homes.

3. What is metabolism?

Metabolism is the entire life cycle, the taking in of nutrients, utilization by the body, and the elimination of waste materials.

4. What are two types of physical fatigue?

Two types of physical fatigue are from overexertion as in exercising too much and underexertion as when one is sick in bed for several days.

5. What can lactic acid buildup cause?

Lactic acid buildup causes the lumps and bumps on the shoulders and also causes fatigue.

6. How can *Shiatsu* help reduce lactic acid buildup?

Shiatsu can apply pressure to the area of the buildup directly to stimulate the circulation and help the body rid itself of the buildup.

7. Why is ambiance important in a *Shiatsu* treatment?

   Ambiance enhances the effectiveness of the treatment and facilitates the relaxation process, hence heightening the effects.

CHAPTER 5

1. Discuss some of the features of one inch of skin.

   One square inch of skin contains: 65 hairs, 95–100 sebaceous glands, 78 yards of nerves, 19 yards of blood vessels, 650 sweat glands, 9,500,000 cells, 1,300 nerve endings to record pain, 19,500 cells at the end of nerve fibers, 78 sensory apparatuses for heat, 13 sensory apparatuses for cold, and 160–165 pressure apparatuses for perception of tactile stimuli.

2. Is a good sense of touch important in *Shiatsu*? Why?

   Yes, it is. A good sense of touch will help you to understand the condition of the body and to know how much pressure to apply to offer an effective treatment. Even though technicians don't diagnose health problems, a good sense of touch helps the technician to understand the body better and indirectly help the client more.

3. What are the primary parts of the body used by the technician to do *Shiatsu*?

   The primary parts of the body used are thumbs, fingers, and palms of hands.

4. How long should pressure be applied and how hard should it be?

   Normally pressure should be applied for about ten seconds depending on the comfort level of the client. The degree of pressure is dependent on the "comfortable pain" threshold of the client. It should never be so hard as to hurt.

5. List a few major contraindications to *Shiatsu*.

   Abdominal area on pregnant person; open wounds; areas of edema, couperose, or varicose veins.

6. Why is it important for the technician to be relaxed when doing a *Shiatsu* treatment?

   It's important for the technician to be relaxed in order to be able to apply the correct amount of pressure in a comfortable, well-timed rhythmic pattern. Also, relaxation helps keep the technician from applying too much pressure.

CHAPTER 6

1. What is the most important factor in client draping?

   The client must be draped so he/she feels very comfortable, safe, secure, and warm. The client in America is generally modest and must not feel exposed.

2. Why is the client consultation chart so important?

   It's important for many reasons with some of the main ones being legal protection to have a record of the client's skin and health state, for marketing to know what products and services have been sold or recommended in the past, and to have a clear understanding of any possible contraindications to treatments.

3. How should the massage table and work area be set up?

   The massage table and work areas must be absolutely immaculate, clean, and neat. Sheets and towels must be fresh, clean, and prepared individually for each client. The table must be sanitized, organized, and orderly.

4. What kind of lighting and music should be used in a *Shiatsu* treatment?

   It's good to have lighting on a rheostat that can be controlled—lighter for consultation and discussion, but with the ability to dim for treatment. Music for *Shiatsu* should be quiet and rhythmic, perhaps offering a slightly oriental theme. Music by Kitaro or similar is ideal for treatments.

5. Why is cleanliness and sanitation so important in treatment?

   Absolute sanitary conditions are critical to give the client a sense of professionalism and safety. Aside from being required, being pristine and clean will further the success rate and confidence a client puts in you and your salon.

6. What kind of massage oil should be used in *Shiatsu*?

   Basically the massage oil should be chosen based on it being very light, nontacky, and not greasy. To have an oriental aura is also esthetically pleasing.

7. Does it matter if the technician has fingernails?

   The technician should never have nails longer than the base of the nail bed. Nails can cut or scratch the client and cause complete failure in applying correct pressure and direction.

8. What aspects of booking clients for treatments are important?

The most important aspect of booking clients for treatments is to be precise in timing. If an hour treatment is booked, that means one hour from arrival to departure.

CHAPTER 7

1. Is massage oil used for facial *Shiatsu* treatments in America?

Yes, a very light massage oil is normally used for treatments. However, if desired, *Shiatsu* can be done without any product.

2. Why would a *Shiatsu* treatment on the head be good to do?

Shiatsu scalp treatments are highly effective for reducing stress and relaxing a client, particularly during the shampoo part of a hair-styling treatment. It really makes the technician stand out and will cause great subsequent success in other *Shiatsu* treatments.

3. How many groups are there in a full facial *Shiatsu* treatment (face, neck, chest)?

There are ten groups of areas in a full facial *Shiatsu* treatment (if you include the closing of hands of the full face): forehead, eyes, nose, cheeks, mouth, full face, ears, neck, shoulders, chest.

4. Normally in a facial treatment, what areas are done with the thumbs?

Temples and shoulders.

5. What does *Shiatsu* in an eye treatment do?

Shiatsu relieves fatigue and stress in the eyes. A headache or redness in the eyes may by accident disappear as well.

CHAPTER 8

1. How long does it take to do *Shiatsu* on the front side of a client and then on the back side if doing a full body treatment?

Thirty-five minutes on the front and twenty-five minutes on the back.

2. Name a few reasons to do *Shiatsu* on the body.

Shiatsu relieves stress in arms and legs and water retention problems in the knees. Circulation of the hands and feet can be greatly improved making the skin better, and increasing nail growth. Stress and tension in the head, chest, and shoulders are relieved by *Shiatsu*.

3. Is it safe to do *Shiatsu* over varicose veins or on a diabetic?

   Shiatsu should not be done on areas of varicose veins. Pressure should be very light on a diabetic because they are so prone to bruising. It may be advisable to obtain a doctor's release to work on areas in question.

4. What is the marketing value of a *Shiatsu* back treatment?

   Everyone loves to have a back rub so adding *Shiatsu* is a great draw into the salon and will help sell *Shiatsu* in other services as well.

5. What good does it do to add *Shiatsu* to a manicure or pedicure?

   Aside from the obvious benefit of relaxation and relief of stress, adding *Shiatsu* makes the treatment more sophisticated and hence, you can charge more for it.

CHAPTER 9

1. Is a good technique sufficient to build the *Shiatsu* business?

   No. Good technique is important, but it's also important to proactively market the new service to build client awareness.

2. How much should you charge for a *Shiatsu* treatment?

   Charges depend on the competition and what the market will bear as well as the per minute value of the technician plus an exotic charge.

3. Why is a brochure or menu important to promote *Shiatsu*?

   Shiatsu must be promoted to build business. The average client doesn't really understand the benefit and the brochure or menu will help bring this awareness.

4. Should you give *Shiatsu* treatments to anyone free?

   Yes, of course. You may want to give some bits of *Shiatsu* free in various salon treatments to introduce the client to the possibility of a full treatment. You would also want to offer the press complimentary treatments.

5. What kind of gift with purchase is good with *Shiatsu*?

   It is good to offer one that is somehow related to the area of the service being done, for example, finishing powder might be nice in a full body treatment. This is also good to offer with package deals as well.

Further Reading

1. Namikoshi, Toru. *The Complete Book of Shiatsu Therapy*. Tokyo, Japan: Japan Publications Inc., 1991.

2. Namikoshi, Toru. *Shiatsu and Stretching*. Tokyo, Japan: Japan Publications Inc., 1992.

3. Mann, Felix. *Acupuncture: The Ancient Art of Healing and How It Works Scientifically*. New York: Vintage Books, A Division of Random House, 1973.

4. Ingham, Eunice D. *Stories The Feet Can Tell*. Florida: Ingham Publishing Inc., 1991.

5. Kunz, Kevin and Barbara. *The Complete Guide to Foot Reflexology*. Englewood Cliffs, NJ: Prentice Hall Inc., 1980.

Bibliography

Bayly, Doreen E. *Reflexology Today: The Stimulation of the Body's Healing Forces through Foot Massage.* Rochester, VT: Healing Arts Press, 1988.

The Burton Goldberg Group. *Alternative Medicine: The Definitive Guide.* Puyallup, WA: Future Medicine Publishing Inc., 1994.

Carter, Mildred & Tammy Weber. *Body Reflexology.* West Nyack, NY: Parker Publishing Co., 1994.

Cerney, J.V. *Acupuncture without Needles.* West Nyack, NY: Parker Publishing Co., 1974.

Chaitow, Leon. *The Acupuncture Treatment of Pain.* Rochester, VT: Healing Arts Press, 1990.

Fitzgerald, William, M.D. & Edwin F. Bowers, M.D. *Handbook of Zone Therapy.* Bombay: D.B. Taraporevala Sons & Co. PVT. LTD., 1986.

Gerson, Joel. *Milady's Standard Textbook for Professional Estheticians.* Albany, NY: Milady Publishing Co., 1992.

Ingham, Eunice D. (With revisions by Dwight C. Byers). *The Original Works of Eunice D. Ingham: Stories the Feet Can Tell through Reflexology, Stories the Feet Have Told through Reflexology.* St. Petersburg, FL: Ingham Publishing, Inc., 1991.

Issel, Christine. *Reflexology: Art, Science, and History.* Sacramento, CA: New Frontier Publishing, 1990.

Kunz, Kevin & Barbara. *The Complete Guide to Foot Reflexology.* Englewood Cliffs, NJ: Prentice Hall Inc., 1980.

———. *Hand and Foot Reflexology: A Self-Help Guide.* New York: Simon & Schuster, 1987.

Lundberg, Paul. *The Book of Shiatsu.* New York: A Fireside Book, Simon & Schuster, 1992.

Mann, Felix. *Acupuncture: The Ancient Art of Healing and How It Works Scientifically.* New York: Vintage Books, a Division of Random House, 1973.

Namikoshi, Tokujiro. *Japanese Finger Pressure Therapy Shiatsu.* Tokyo: Japan Publications Inc., 1975.

Namikoshi, Toru. *The Complete Book of Shiatsu Therapy.* Tokyo: Japan Publications Inc., 1991.

———. *Shiatsu and Stretching.* Tokyo: Japan Publications Inc., 1985, 1992.

———. *Shiatsu Therapy Theory and Practice.* Tokyo: Japan Publications Inc., 1974.

Serizawa, M.D. Kstsuseke. *Massage: The Oriental Method.* Tokyo: Japan Publications, Inc., 1972.

Shultz, William. *Shiatsu Japanese Finger Pressure Therapy.* New York: Bell Publishing Co., 1976.

Tappan, Frances M. *Healing Massage Techniques.* Reston, VA: Reston Publishing Co., A Prentice Hall Company, 1978.

Yamamoto, Shizuko. *Barefoot Shiatsu.* Tokyo: Japan Publications Inc., 1979.

Glossary/Index

Note: Page numbers in **bold** indicate art figures.

A

Abdomen, **99**, 99-100
Acupuncture, needle insertion into the body at strategic points,
     6-7, 17
Advertising, 120-121
Ambiance of room, 39-40, 60-62
Amma massage, 25, 45
Appointment book, 67
Arm treatment, 94-96, **95-98**, 109-110
Auriculotherapy, 18
Ayurvedic medicine, system combining natural therapies with a
     highly personalized approach to the treatment of disease, 5

B

Back side *Shiatsu,* 100-108, **102-107**
Back treatment, 104, 106, **106-107**, 108-109
Becke, Robert O., 18
Body *Shiatsu,* 89-111
Bowers, Edwin, 15
Byers, Dwight, 16

C

Carter, Mildred, 16
Chest *Shiatsu,* 99-100, **99-100**
Chi. See Ki
Chinese medicine, 6-8
Client, handling, 67-68
Client consultation chart, 62-64
Clocks, 61
Color schemes, 60
Conception vessel, 26
Cornelius, Alfons, 14

D

Darwin, Charles, 11

M

Mailings, 118
Marketing services, 115–122
Massage table setup, 64
Meissner's corpuscles, common receptors for light touch that are located in the dermis, 47
Mental fatigue, exhaustion from emotional overload or highly active mental work, 37
Meridian system, 17–18
Metabolism, the taking in of nutrients, utilization by the body of the important substances, and the elimination of waste materials, 38
Mind/body harmony, 36
Modern Zone Therapy, 15
Moxibustion, 6
Music, 62

N

Namikoshi, Tokujiro, 9, 16
Neck treatment
  back, 104, **105**
  front, 99–100, **99–100**
Nei Ching, 6-7
Nippon Shiatsu School, 9, 16
Nogier, Paul, 18

O

Oils, 60, 65

P

Pacinian corpuscles, encapsulated endings normally located between the dermis and subcutaneous layer that are receptors for deeper pressure, 47
Pain relief, 32
Palm pressure
  inner, **52**
  outer, **52**
  overlapping, **53**
Palms, 51
Partial service *Shiatsu,* 115–116
Physical fatigue, extreme under- or overexertion using the physical body, 37

Notes

Notes

Notes

Notes

Notes

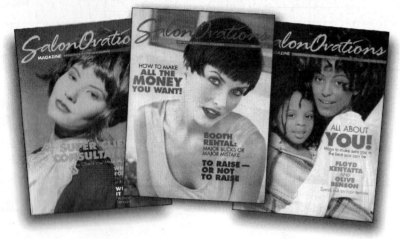
Notes

_____
_____
_____
_____
_____
_____
_____
_____
_____
_____
_____
_____
_____
_____
_____
_____
_____
_____
_____
_____
_____
_____
_____
_____

Notes

_____

_____

_____

_____

_____

_____

_____

_____

_____

_____

_____

_____

_____

_____

_____

_____

_____

_____

_____

_____

Notes

_____

_____

_____

_____

_____

_____

_____

_____

_____

_____

_____

_____

_____

_____

_____

_____

_____

_____

_____

_____